CONTENTS

GUIDE FOR HOUSE SURGEONS
IN THE
SURGICAL UNIT

SEVENTH EDITION

G. J. Fraenkel

M.A., B.M., M.Ch. (Oxon.), F.R.C.S., F.R.A.C.S., F.R.A.C.M.A.

Foundation Dean, School of Medicine, Flinders University, South Australia. Former Ralph Barnett Professor of Surgery in the University of Otago, Dunedin, New Zealand. Former Surgical Tutor, The Radcliffe Infirmary, Oxford. Former Member, Court of Examiners Royal Australasian College of Surgeons.

J. Ludbrook

B.Med.Sc., M.D., Ch.M. (N.Z.), F.R.C.S., F.R.A.C.S.

Associate Director and N.H. & M.R.C. Senior Principal Research Fellow, Baker Medical Research Institute, Melbourne, Australia. Former Dorothy Mortlock Professor of Surgery, University of Adelaide. Former Professor of Surgery, University of New South Wales. Former Senior Lecturer in Surgery, University of Otago. Member of Council and former Chairman, Board of Examiners, Royal Australasian College of Surgeons.

H. A. F. Dudley

Ch.M. (Edin.), F.R.C.S., F.R.C.S. (Edin.), F.R.A.C.S.

Professor of Surgery, St. Mary's Hospital Medical School, London, England. Former Foundation Professor of Surgery, Monash University, Melbourne, Australia. Former Senior Lecturer in Surgery, University of Aberdeen, Scotland.

G. L. Hill

M.D. (Leeds), Ch.M. (Otago), F.R.C.S., F.R.A.C.S.

Professor and Chairman, Department of Surgery, University of Auckland, New Zealand. Former Reader in Surgery, University of Leeds, England.

V. R. Marshall

M.D., F.R.A.C.S.

Director of Urology, Flinders Medical Centre, Associate Professor of Surgery, Flinders University of South Australia. Senior Visiting Transplant Surgeon, Queen Elizabeth Hospital; Senior Specialist, Repatriation General Hospital; Consultant in Urology, The Royal Adelaide Hospital, Australia.

WILLIAM HEINEMANN MEDICAL BOOKS LTD.
LONDON

First published 1961
Second revised Edition 1962
Third Edition 1964
Fourth Edition 1968
Reprinted 1971
Fifth Edition 1974
Sixth Edition 1978
Seventh Edition 1982

ISBN 0-433-10803-7

Photoset in VIP Times
by D. P. Media Limited,
Hitchin, Hertfordshire
Printed and bound by
Redwood Burn Ltd, Trowbridge
and Melksham, Wiltshire

ii

PREFACE TO THE SEVENTH EDITION

This guide has its origin in loose leaf folders of notes which were provided to help house surgeons on the Professorial Surgical Unit at the Dunedin Hospital, Dunedin, New Zealand. The fact that these notes frequently disappeared plus other indications of a wider demand resulted in the publication of the Guide to House Surgeons in the Surgical Unit by the University Book Shop Ltd., Dunedin, in 1961, followed by a second revised edition in 1962. Since then the work seems to have acquired a life of its own.

The requirements of different clinicians vary considerably with regard to the recording of case histories and findings on physical examination, the selection of special investigations and pre- and post-operative management. Nevertheless there is sufficient common ground in general surgery to justify a guide such as this. Its aim is to standardise various aspects of the investigation and management of patients suffering from a variety of common surgical conditions. Whenever possible, an explanation of the reasons behind a particular routine is provided. When certain investigations seem obscure and when no explanation is given, they have been included for the purpose of some specific study.

In addition to the points which are covered with regard to particular disorders, some general topics are discussed to enable you to get the maximum work done in the minimum of time.

Everywhere that we have had the good fortune to work, we have found common threads running through the way surgical patients are cared for, however much the 'house rules' may vary between individual institutions. It is this, and the fact that our little guide keeps disappearing from the booksellers shelves, which has encouraged us to keep the volume going.

We are conscious that the term 'house surgeon' embraces 'housemen' and 'housewomen'. Because the latter sobriquet may still, in our unenlightened age, carry the connotation of housewife, we have persisted with the chauvinistic 'houseman' and the general epithet 'he'. This is not to underestimate in any way those housewomen who have in both professional and social ways lightened our task and provided a disproportionate amount of the cement that holds good units together.

G. J. Fraenkel, Adelaide; J. Ludbrook, Melbourne;
H. A. F. Dudley, London; G. L. Hill, Auckland;
V. R. Marshall, Adelaide

1982

ACKNOWLEDGEMENTS

In preparing this revision we have been joined by two younger men who not only bring special skills in their own fields, but also have had a very broad experience of surgery in general. In addition, we have had the benefit of detailed criticism and advice solicited from and proffered by colleagues from around the world: Prof. C. J. Alexander; Prof. G. T. Benness; Prof. J. P. Blandy; Dr A. J. C. Bune; Prof. A. Cuschieri; Mr H. B. Devlin; Dr R. B. Ellis-Pegler; Mr I. B. Faris; Mr J. Fitzsimons; Dr G. A. Foote; Prof. I. E. Gillespie; Dr R. Hecker; Dr A. J. Irving; Prof. K. E. F. Hobbs; Prof. M. Hobsley; Mr G. G. Jamieson; Prof. I. D. A. Johnston; Mr C. R. Kapadia; Dr S. L. P. Langlois; Mr P. J. Lyndon; Mr T. J. McNair; Dr M. A. Marion; Det. Supt. C. F. Payne; Assoc. Prof. J. C. Probert; Dr D. L. Rothwell; Dr W. J. Russell; Prof. D. Shearman; Prof. R. Shields; Prof. A. G. Wangel; Dr. J. A. Whitworth; Dr D. G. Woodfield.

Mr H. Brendan Devlin has very kindly collated and enlarged on the material on forensic problems.

1. ADMINISTRATION

The Houseman's Role

A houseman occupies a unique position in the team of those who are looking after surgical inpatients. His role is complex, yet he is ill-prepared for it by those theoretical aspects of his undergraduate examinations upon which his teachers have exhorted him to concentrate. At one and the same time he is expected to be an organiser (getting patients from place to place, arranging their investigation and treatment), a scribe (keeping records and filling in forms), a guide and counsellor (seeing relatives and talking at length to patients about their problems), a minor executive (undertaking practical procedures), and an unfailing source of information to his senior colleagues on all aspects of those under his care. The diversified job specification is a daunting one, but at the same time it is the fastest way of bringing the new doctor to clinical maturity. He will get there quicker if he understands that the hospital is a very complex organisation, the structure of which he must master if he is to use its potential for the care of his patients.

A hospital can be looked upon as a set of discrete areas, each under separate control, all ostensibly there for the good of the patient, but all functioning largely independently of each other. The connections between them are made by the communication of data about patients and the passage of those individuals who have roles in more than one place from area to area. Prominent as both a communicator and as a man who gyrates between operating theatre, ward, outpatients and special departments, is the houseman. His success will be directly proportional to his basic understanding of how to communicate, how to arrange for things to be done to (and for) his patients, and to his being obvious as an individual who is prepared to exert himself in seeing that communication is not impersonal. To achieve the one he must rapidly come to grips with the technical details of which forms to fill in, which days to choose for certain investigations, which individual to approach for a given purpose. In this he may be assisted by whatever local manual is produced by the hospital in which he is working, but such manuals are far from commonplace and usually he must pick up his skills in this field entirely by word of mouth. To acquire success in personal contact it is necessary to devote time and thought to the process; five minutes spent in taking an X-ray request slip down to the department with a courteous verbal expansion of the details that have been written down, and a similar time devoted to delivering the theatre list in person to the reputedly draconian theatre superintendent, pay dividends out of all proportion to the effort involved. Failing a personal appearance, care should always be taken in the wording of the request or list. Often these are badly written: not only illegible, but also not conveying what the *problem* is or what exactly are the intentions of the surgical team. Always write out a request in terms of what is expected from the examination, not merely as a bald statement of what the patient is thought to have wrong with him. Finally, judicious use of the telephone to supplement the written word can be helpful, but it must be remembered that for a houseman to call a very senior colleague requires a well-developed sense of tact.

The houseman should also not forget the informal communication network which exists in every organisation and is a particular feature of hospitals. More can often be accomplished by knowing and being on good terms with secretaries, porters, orderlies, and administrators than by cultivating the more Olympian members of the medical profession. Paramedical and non-medical personnel make up the skeleton of function upon which the flesh of nursing and medicine is hung. Their very permanence gives them a knowledge and authority which can be most useful if properly exploited and very humiliating if it is used to make the houseman feel inferior. Their friendly advice should rarely, if ever, be neglected.

Finally, one of the hardest things to learn about a hospital is that it is a place of tension. There is tension in the ill patient; the tension among those who worry about making him well (and also about the views of others as to their competence); the tension of long hours and irregular sleep patterns; and last, and perhaps most regrettably, the stress of an organisation that is too hierarchically organised. Many of these things are changing, but it is well to remember that when there are inexplicable rows, unworthy assignment of blame, and seemingly irrational behaviour, the human situation described may be the cause. As the bottom man on the totem pole, the wise house surgeon will not only scorn delights and live laborious days, but also keep his head even if all about him others are losing theirs. If he is wise he will be quiet in his comments and neutral in his attitudes.

Some Practical Points

1. Keep a notebook and write *everything* down, crossing it off as you do it. Don't use the back of envelopes.

2. Try to get order into your day so that you are doing the same thing at the same time.

3. Think ahead all the time—who is going home, who needs social care, who might be going to the operating room.

4. Always reflect before you act whether or not you should inform someone else—the usual answer is that you should.

5. Make sure that your immediate associates know what to do and when you need to know.

6. Arrange investigations on patients so that the results will provide

(a) diagnostic decisions as soon as possible

(b) baseline for surgical management at the appropriate moment.

Admissions

All patients must be seen at the earliest possible opportunity and notes written up forthwith. Construct an investigation plan for every patient (see Records, below). Some tests may have been done or ordered from the Outpatients Department for those who are being routinely admitted. Others may be suggested in the notes. The following are useful guides. *All* patients who are destined for major surgery should have the following investigations at least considered:

Weight and height

Ward urinalysis

Full haematologic screen (blood count, examination of a film)

Biochemical screen (including electrolytes and blood urea) for abdominal surgery

Chest X-ray in patients over the age of 30 who have not had a chest X-ray in the last year and/or have respiratory symptoms.

In some hospitals:

Nose and throat swabs

Sickle cell solubility test in black patients

All patients over the age of 40 who are to undergo major surgery should, if resources permit, have a standard ECG done.

In any patient in whom respiratory problems exist or in whom thoracotomy is contemplated, obtain:

Sputum culture
Vital capacity and forced vital capacity in one second (FEV_1)
(before and after bronchodilators)
Arterial pO_2 and pCO_2

Remember that consultations with others may be required at, or shortly after, the time of admission and if days are not to be wasted these should be set up at once. This is particularly true of the need to look after the psychosocial side of the patient, who may be more worried about wages or family care than about his illness.

Later in this Guide there are details of differential diagnosis to consider, and further investigations to undertake, in specific surgical conditions or situations.

Patients who are admitted as a matter of *emergency* present special problems, dealt with under individual headings. However, they may have a past history of surgical or other treatment elsewhere. It is not adequate to accept their version of such an episode—wherever possible you must aim to get the information direct by using the telephone to contact the records office of the previous hospital or the general practitioner concerned.

Records

Most doctors do not enjoy keeping records. Yet time and time again the usefulness of past information to current management can be clearly demonstrated. Surprisingly, in spite of all such examples, we are still far from agreeing what should be recorded and how. Most conventional hospital records are dry as dust, little used as a day-to-day method of handling the patient's course, and often deficient in the items of information posterity wants. It it little wonder that the houseman senses a lack of interest from his seniors in the whole matter of record keeping. How then are we to preserve the good and necessary features of records, and at the same time generate enthusiasm for their completion?

One answer to this question lies in the use of what it has become fashionable to call 'problem orientation'. The conventional information on history and physical examination is collected as before, but it is used merely as a matrix against which all those concerned attempt to define a list of problems which confront the patient. Management and the recording of progress is then conducted with reference to this list, adding or subtracting to and from it as occasion demands and as new problems appear or old ones become inactive. The value of this approach is that the record becomes a dynamic vehicle for communication and there is usually also a much clearer delineation of the exact way in which the patient should be handled.

Problem orientation must start with the house surgeon who makes the initial problem list but it cannot end there; he is not alone in the exercise. If he is to make a record work in this way he must insist, cajole, wheedle or inveigle others into putting down their thoughts in concrete terms. Similarly in the surgical setting, operation notes are not very useful unless they are preceded by an explanation of *why* surgery was undertaken and contain in their text the argument why a certain course of action was chosen. This is particularly the case if they are part of the means of communication with the patient's doctor outside hospital.

The future of problem orientation in medical records is not exactly clear. In the meantime it is recommended as the basic way a record should be kept and particularly how the progress notes should be arranged. A brief example is shown below. As with many things, this is just an ordering and rationalising of what already happens, but with the advantage of leaving a clearer account of what actually took place for those who may have to scan the record and draw conclusions about the patient either in your absence or at some future date.

Postoperative progress Mr H. F.

Problem List
>   1. Partial gastrectomy for DU.
>   2. Preoperative chronic bronchitis
>   3. Anxiety state.

Day 1. 1. Bowel sounds absent. Duodenal stump drain 90 ml. Nil orally; for gastrografin swallow tomorrow to see if oral feeding can begin.
>   2. Some coarse rales at right base. Chest X-ray shows increased hilar density only, without evidence of collapse-consolidation. Continue preoperative

physiotherapy. No indication for antibiotics at time but repeat physical examination and X-ray tomorrow.

       3. Reaction to operation less acute than expected. Continue diazepam 2 mg IM for next 24 hours on same schedule as preoperatively (6 hourly).

Day 2. 1. Bowel sounds present. Gastrografin shows contrast in terminal ileum at one hour. Begin oral fluids.

       2. Chest sounds less and X-ray *not* taken. *Note by physiotherapist*—he is doing well but his sputum remains thick and he is wheezy intermittently; would bronchodilators be helpful? Thanks, yes we will prescribe.

       3. No change. Consider withdrawing diazepam tomorrow but remember that he may have difficulty in sleeping.

Indeed there is much to be said for a single record used by everyone. This example includes one excellent feature of the problem orientated record namely that it is not exclusive to the medical profession as records have tended to be in the past.

Responsibility

It is difficult to lay down a clear division of responsibility within a unit, but the following general principle applies: if you are worried about a patient or some unforeseen complication arises, examine the patient as fully as possible and then *tell* your immediate senior—it then becomes *his* concern, and *his* responsibility as to whether he should see the patient or not. Likewise *tell* whoever is responsible for the emergency surgery of all emergency admissions as soon as you have examined them. A particular problem which often gives rise to confusion is when a patient is transferred to a specialist unit—e.g. the Intensive Care Unit—during his hospital stay. Such units usually have their own house staff and routines and expect you to let them take responsibility for writing orders, drugs and fluid balances. This makes it difficult for you to maintain continuity in your care. Though it adds to your work load you *must* keep abreast of what is going on because if you do not the patient may suffer from the other team's lack of knowledge of what you know. When responsibility is handed back you will be out of touch.

Last, let us set a question to all potential housemen. If you have just gone to bed at 2 a.m. after a hard day and the night nurse calls to say she is worried about Mrs Brown, what is your answer? For those of us who believe in responsibility in medicine there can be only one—'I'll be up to see her within 5 minutes.'

Ward Routine

Find out from the Ward Sister what is the most convenient time for you to do your daily round with her or the duty nurse. Also, ask what are the meal times and any other periods when it will not be possible for the nursing staff to accompany you, unless it is an emergency. It is unreasonable to arrive on the ward to see a non-acutely ill patient in the middle of dinner and then be cross because no one pays any attention to you.

Consultations

The transfer of responsibility or the request for advice is one of the most delicate matters in medicine. With increasing specialisation in the technology of care, there is all too often the tendency to call in an 'expert' who will deal with a part of the patient but not the whole. To avoid this unsatisfactory situation the request is usually made to a senior member of the Unit to be consulted in the belief that he will concern himself overall with the patient. Each hospital has its own method of setting up this situation so that protocol is respected and propriety not offended. It is wise for housemen and registrars to undertake informal liaison at the same time as a more formal approach is being made; this permits some prior knowledge of what the consulted person is likely to expect in the way of attendance by a member of the team, special investigations, or arrangements for him to examine the patient in some particular way. Whether you transmit the formal request verbally (or, as it more usual and preferable, in writing) it is best, unless you are specifically instructed to the contrary, to make it a *request for an opinion*. In writing a request it should be in plain English, should avoid unnecessary details that can be obtained from the records, and should specify the problem for which the consultation has been requested. When more than an opinion is asked for, ascertain from one of the other and more senior members of your team what are the exact terms of reference—advice about some particular aspect of the patient, or to take over the management of the whole matter. When the matter is urgent by all means speak to the consultant concerned over the telephone, but it is a good thing to reflect whether such an approach might come better from someone else higher in the pecking order!

For ENT, eye and some other opinions where special equipment is needed it may be more convenient for the patient to attend the appropriate Outpatient Clinic.

Relatives

On all occasions you should be friendly and helpful to a patient's relatives, particularly when the patient is a minor.

It is also important always to discover the precise degree of relationship, so that information is not given which might lead to subsequent difficulties. This situation occasionally arises with patients in whom for instance pregnancy or veneral disease is suspected or established.

With this proviso, it is one of your important duties to make sure that relatives are kept informed as to the nature of the diagnosis, likely operations, prognosis, or any deterioration in the patient's condition. When a patient's condition unexpectedly deteriorates, or a patient is to undergo an operation the outcome of which is uncertain, it is vital that a member of the unit informs the relatives in person or by telephone.

Close relatives who express a wish to do so are fully entitled to see the surgeon in charge of the case, and you may make an appointment for them to do so. You will find also that in some instances the surgeon himself will express a wish to see the relatives, and this is arranged as a rule to take place during or immediately after a ward round or outpatient session.

Difficulties may arise because the information given to patients and relatives by different members of the team either is, or appears to be, inconsistent. An active house surgeon will take the initiative as co-ordinator of what has been said.

The Referring Doctor

It is important to remember that the patient's family doctor has entrusted the patient to your hospital unit for *specialised surgical care*. He will continue to be the physician and counsellor to the patient and his family when the former leaves hospital. At the very least, he must be informed within a very short time of the patient's discharge from hospital about the more important features of the *diagnosis*, *treatment*, and of *recommendations for further care*. If it is important that the patient consult him shortly after leaving hospital, both he and the patient should be informed. He must receive an accurate account of any *drugs* or other forms of treatment with which the patient should continue once he returns home. If a detailed written account of these matters cannot reach the family doctor within 48 hours, he should be given the necessary information by telephone or by a brief summary which accompanies or precedes the patient.

If the patient should die in hospital, it is important that his family doctor be informed within a matter of hours: it may be he to whom the family turns for information and advice.

The Patient

It is an unusual person who is not disturbed by his admission to hospital. He may be more or less greatly distressed by the unfamiliar and often *frightening environment*, by the uncertainties which surround an *operation*, by fears regarding his *physical ailment*, and by anxieties in regard to his *domestic life or work*. The surgical resident plays a vital role in all these aspects of the patient's illness. Because of his frequent attendance on the patient he is often looked upon overtly or covertly by the patient as a counsellor. He fails in his duty if he does not spend the time which is necessary to explain the patient's illness to him, explain the circumstances which will surround his operation and the postoperative period, and recognise and attempt to alleviate any other source of distress to the patient.

The particular stresses to which surgical patients are exposed may sometimes lead to bizarre behaviour. Some patients become passive, apathetic and depressed; others aggressive and truculent; yet others excited and even occasionally disorientated. Normal traits such as obsessiveness may become exaggerated. Complete denial of the illness may occur. It is very important that the houseman recognises the possibility that the patient's behaviour is not normal, and that he takes this into consideration both in designing treatment (e.g. sedation) and in providing commonsense psychological counsel, (see also Acute Postoperative Mental Disturbance, p. 106). The reactions of patients to hospital admission are also culturally based. Care must be taken not to assume that what appears odd to you is abnormal to the patient.

Particular problems arise in patients who have cancer or are dying. In the past it has often been the custom to conceal the facts from the patient by the use of euphemism or tactics of denial which amount to untruth. As often as not this is misguided. In those who have firm faith of a religious kind, or who are well supported by close family ties or by friends, a conspiracy of silence can do more harm than good and frequently involves the medical staff and patient in contortions of evasion ultimately resulting in a loss of mutual confidence when, as it will, the truth comes out. The general axiom is that the truth, well put and hedged around with the appropriate and real uncertainties that must accompany any attempt to foretell death or disaster, should be the usual strategy. The exception is the lonely, self-supporting individual who has already shown strong denial mechanisms towards his illness.

The tactics used in bringing a patient to grips with a diagnosis such as cancer which is threatening to him, or with the finality of death, can only be cultivated by experience; clearly no doctor in his right senses bluntly and baldly puts the facts before his patient. As with other interviews it is best to encourage the patient to talk about his illness: sometimes it is clear from such preliminary skirmishing that denial is a strong force and no further action should be taken, nor has harm been done; sometimes it is immediately apparent that he knows or suspects and is anxious to talk the matter over. The recognition of the serious nature of the situation by the patient should lead the houseman to move on quickly to considering the positive side of the matter—how plans should be made and what physical and financial support can be arranged. Before talking to a patient about problems of cancer, death and disablement you should have discussed the matter not only with your medical seniors so that all are aware of the plan, but also with those who are going to help solve social and family problems. It is increasingly clear that the social worker is vital in the management of many situational crises of this kind and the houseman must learn from the outset how to work with her for the good of his patients. It is not enough to identify the possibility of a social problem, write a request for consultation by the social worker and then forget the matter in the hurly-burly of acute surgical action. The unique position of the houseman in relation to his patients gives him an understanding of facts and attitudes useful to the social worker

10

and makes it necessary that he should be seen to be concerned as part of the team solving these problems. Again, cultural differences must be borne in mind. We all now live in a polyglot society and must understand our neighbours' differences as never before.

On the rare occasions when a patient asks directly if he has cancer or is dying, it is a legal obligation to give an answer which to the best of your belief is true. It is also important to give a clear explanation of diagnosis and prognosis to the patient's closest relatives, but it is not usually helpful, or indeed fair, to ask them to make the decision on what the patient should be told, however much you must draw them into the business of telling.

When it has been agreed to discuss matters of this kind with the patient or when he demands information, the facts and their outcome should always be recorded in the notes. Apart from being a basic part of the medical record, this avoids uncertainty for others in the future, especially when the patient returns and says 'doctor said it wasn't cancer' or 'nobody told me anything'.

There are two problems which precede death. The first is caused by the presence in most hospitals of a cardiac arrest team. If they are to do their job effectively they must act rapidly and without debate. Thus they cannot easily pause to discriminate over the rights and wrongs of resuscitating an individual patient. It follows that the surgeons and nurses must, however distasteful it seems to be, discuss who should and who should not be resuscitated. In some institutions this also means writing in the record that a patient is or is not 'for resuscitation'. The important matter is that the house surgeon must be absolutely clear about how to proceed, even if he has to badger his seniors to get a definite answer.

The second matter is organ donation. The needs of the individual and the relatives must be balanced against the needs of others. No one wants to deny health and survival to the patient with chronic renal failure or irremediable cardiac disease. Equally, no one wants to confront the relatives of (say) a decerebrate patient with the imminence of death. However, the reality of life and death has to be faced. The houseman must be alert to the possibility of 'potential donors' and thus to put into action whatever local procedures exist. These will include certain approaches that have to be made to the relatives and the transplant team and baseline investigations on the patient. You should be sure about local arrangements so you are not caught unawares (see also p. 189).

Deaths

It is important that you notify all deaths to the immediate senior member of the staff responsible for the patient; at once in the case of unexpected death and as soon as is reasonable in predicted deaths.

Surgical units have sometimes been judged by the assiduity with which they seek and secure autopsies. This is admirable, but can be carried to ridiculous and painful lengths. A more enlightened attitude is to debate each instance on its merits, starting from the premise that reasons must be found for *not* having an autopsy. Autopsies are *your* direct responsibility, and if deaths occur when you are off duty, on your return you must check that permission has been sought. One should endeavour to ensure that a patient does not leave the ward until all arrangements have been made.

In certain circumstances a death must be reported to the *coroner*. The rules vary in different parts of the world and even, for instance between England and Scotland. In England and in many other countries: deaths in the operating theatre; deaths following (at whatever remove) accident or suspected crime; and unexpected deaths in a wide variety of circumstances must be reported. If certain words such as 'alcohol' appear on a death certificate, the death is automatically referred to the coroner. The coroner's office is almost always a helpful institution and a phone call is the best way of discussing any problem. You must consult if you are to avoid getting caught in a sandwich between your seniors and the coroner.

Outpatient Follow-up

In most units it is an invariable rule that every patient be seen at least once after his leaving hospital, in the outpatient clinic of the surgeon who carried out the operation or who was responsible for the investigation. This appointment should be for 2 to 3 weeks after leaving hospital, unless other instructions are given.

After one postoperative visit, many patients need not be seen again, and the patient and his family doctor should be informed of this. However, in most units patients with certain diseases will be followed up for very much longer periods. This is often true of patients with malignant disease; of patients with other diseases in which the unit is conducting a special study; or where for other reasons it is the patient's interest to be seen regularly by a specialist surgeon.

Prescribing

Prescribe precisely and you will benefit your patients, save money and stay out of trouble.

1. *Use the approved name*—the proprietary name may be added in parentheses. Some authorities now question this view because proprietaries vary in their potency and availability, but we continue to support it.

2. *Specify the dosage*—not just as '1 tablet t.d.s' but as '0.5g tablets 1 t.d.s.'

3. *Specify the route*—injections should be specified as IM or SC.

4. *Specify the duration of treatment*—whenever this is possible and always with antibiotics. On all patients check the prescription list every 24 hours and ask if particular drugs need to be continued. On complex problems insist on a 'therapy review' every three or four days, to be undertaken by all concerned.

Medicine and the Law

In hospital practice the law impinges on medicine in three main areas: professional negligence, confidentiality, and certification. Both the law and its interpretation may differ substantially between one country and another, between state and state in countries where such devolution exists and may vary even from one city to another in the same state. In any case of doubt therefore you should always consult one of the administrative officers of the hospital, because in the majority of cases the hospital will also be involved in any medico-legal matter that is of concern to you.

The most important piece of advice *in regard to professional negligence* is that you should at all times carry the best insurance policy you can afford against claims for professional negligence, whether or not the hospital is also insured. The hospital's insurers will safeguard the interests of the hospital, which may conflict with your own. Many cases of alleged professional negligence are hard or impossible to defend because adequate records are not available. Let this be an additional incentive to you for keeping the fullest possible account.

13

You should also spend one of your spare free evenings in reading the annual reports of some of these insurance companies. They are often entertaining and instructive.

In regard to confidentiality there are certain easy guidelines. It is unwise to discuss a patient's case over the telephone and very much better to speak to the enquirer in person after it has been established that the patient wishes you to communicate the information, or that the enquirer is entitled to the information by virtue of a very close relationship. You must insist on having a signed consent form from the patient or his legal guardian before providing a written report about his medical condition to anyone except his personal medical attendants. All enquiries from the press about patients should be referred to the hospital administration.

In regard to certification read carefully any prescription or document which you sign and be sure that you hold all the qualifications necessary to sign such a document in that particular city. Be very sure to distinguish between fact and opinion, and never sign a document stating that you have carried out a certain examination or other procedure when in fact this is not the case. When there is any doubt whatever, consult an officer of the hospital or your professional insurance company, or both. The matter of the certification of death presents great difficulties at any time, and never more so than when the issue of the donation of an organ for transplantation arises. The law and the practice of coroners and coroner's offices is so varied that it is essential for you to seek instruction as to the types of deaths of which the local coroner likes notification and the form in which he likes it. For instance, in some areas all cases of jaundice as the cause of death are automatically notified to the coroner because of past records of industrial poisoning in that town. You must study the preferences of the local coroner in regard to death certification, because in most countries a coroner has such very wide discretion that a coroner who dislikes the way you handle things can make your life very miserable indeed.

(Forensic problems, see p. 196 *et seq*.)

2. MANAGEMENT OF OPERATIONS

Order of Operation Lists

Three factors should govern this:

1. Though in theory the way the theatre is run, and the ventilation should make it possible for a 'septic' patient to precede a 'clean' one with impunity, in real life this is not so. There are several studies which attest to the higher incidence of sepsis the further down the list a clean case is found. Therefore arrange clean before dirty.

2. A patient for whom something outside the theatre is required (e.g. a frozen section or an operative cholegram) should be scheduled at a set time (usually the beginning of a list or after a first operation of highly predictable duration). This always helps smooth external relations.

3. It is a good idea to start with a small operation of fixed duration which allows a 'warm up' period and which gives the theatre staff a chance to set up for a longer and more complicated case at leisure.

4. If (a), (b) and (c) can be achieved, it is a good thing to give the more elderly surgeon – fixed in his ways and even sometimes quite busy – a chance to start at a set time.

The operation list that goes to the theatre should specify:
(a) the procedure
(b) the approach (e.g., transabdominal, transthoracic)
(c) the position of the patient if it is to be unusual (e.g., Lloyd Davis)
(d) any extras required (e.g., catheterisation)
(e) extra procedures (e.g., radiology)

The house-surgeon is advised to go through the check lists which follow for each patient before and after operation. Some of the items are then discussed in more detail.

Preoperative Check List

While the details of making the arrangements for a patient to be operated on vary from hospital to hospital, the house surgeon's responsibility is usually clear: to make sure that no essential steps in the process have been omitted. Most hospitals have a system, but

15

most systems require the very active collaboration of the house surgeon.

The following is a list of items that the house surgeon should check for each patient who is to go to the operating room.

Has the *surgeon* been consulted about the patient or list of patients?

Has *theatre* been notified of the list, and does the list contain an accurate description of the intended *operation* and all that is needed for it?

Has the *patient* had the operation and early postoperative course, explained to him? Is it necessary or desirable to consult with his relatives?

Is a stoma contemplated? (See p. 159.)

Has the formal *consent* form for operation been properly completed?

Are the baseline investigations in order and within normal limits?

Has the patient any *allergies* or *hypersensitivities*?

e.g. Antibiotics
　　　Anaesthetics
　　　Applications (e.g. iodine, adhesive plaster)

Is the patient on any *drugs* that should either be stopped or their route of administration changed?

e.g. Antihypertensives
　　　Antidepressants
　　　Anticoagulants

Does the patient require any new or additional *medication*?

e.g. Diabetic control
　　　Antibiotics
　　　Steroids

Has the *anaesthetist* been notified?

Does the *Ward Sister* know which of her patients are to be operated on?

Special preoperative orders for patients—

　　　Area to be *shaved*
　　　Nasogastric tube?
　　　IV infusion?
　　　Urethral catheter?

16

Any *special requirements* for the operation—
  Blood cross match?
  Peroperative *radiography*?
  Frozen section histopathology?
  Clinical *photography*?

Any foreseeable *postoperative* requirements?
  Intensive care accommodation
  Physiotherapy

Immediate Postoperative Check List

Before you and the patient leave the operating theatre, a number of matters must be attended to:

Make sure that *biopsy* or *operation specimens* are properly packaged, (*e.g. histological material in the right fixative, bacteriological material in the right transport medium*), labelled, and accompanied by a request form
Make sure an *operation note* is completed (at least in summary, if it is to be typed in full later)
Check with surgeon and anaesthetist re *immediate postoperative instructions:*
  Pain relief
  IV or oral intake
  Nursing observations required
  Management of tubes, drains, catheters
  Any special drugs, e.g. antibiotics

General Notes and Checks on Postoperative Management

Daily Check List

Temperature, pulse, respiration: is there any untoward trend? If so why?
Fluid intake and output (urine and drains)?
Are orders (including fluid orders) up to date?
Have the appropriate tests been ordered for the next day (always complete forms the evening before at the latest)?
Can the patient take drugs by mouth that are at present being given parenterally?

17

Should antibiotics be stopped?

Are sutures ready for removal? In general:

(a) Clips are removed from the neck on day 2 and from other sites on days 5–7

(b) Sutures are removed from the neck and face on day 2 and from the abdomen on days 7–10

Is/are drain(s) ready for removal? In general drains that have been inserted for:

> *Blood*, are left 36–48 hours
>
> *Chest drainage after thoracotomy*, are left until a chest X-ray confirms full expansion, and drainage is less than 100ml day
>
> *Suture lines* are left for 5–7 days
>
> *Pus* are left until there is no further drainage and/or a sinogram fails to show a residual cavity

N.B. a tube inserted transabdominally into the gastro-intestinal tract (gastrostomy, jejunostomy. T-tube drainage of the biliary tree) should be left for a minimum of 8 days—i.e. until it is unequivocally sealed off from the peritoneal cavity.

Biochemical management. Serum electrolyte concentrations after operation, while useful as a check on normality, are no certain method of ensuring that all is well. They tend to be done daily but unless the situation is changing rapidly, every second day is quite adequate. Once parenteral therapy has been stopped there is rarely any need to make further measurements unless the clinical context suggests something amiss. Urine electrolyte levels, combined with a knowledge of urine volume, are very useful in checking balance and are not done often enough. They are essential in assessing repletion of a potassium-deficient patient.

Haemoglobin should be checked in the 3rd postoperative day in any patient who has had major blood loss at the time of accident or operation, and twice weekly in patients with sepsis or making a complicated postoperative recovery.

Suspicion of sepsis (see Temperature Charts on p. 114). Examine the wound for tenderness, redness or discharge. Culture every available secretion. Take a blood culture and repeat until two consecutive cultures are negative. Have a blood film examined at the earliest possible opportunity for the presence of toxic granulations and/or Doehle bodies. Consult on the appropriate antibiotic regimen and other investigations (see also patients on long term parenteral nutrition p. 82).

Patients on intravenous therapy. Check the IV site of all patients daily. Tenderness at the infusion point is an indication to change it. With or without this, intravenous infusions should ideally not run for more than 24 hours at one site.

Patients with indwelling catheters should have a urine culture every third day.

Removing drains and other minor procedures on the postoperative patient (see also p. 24). When a drain is to be removed or an *open* wound dressed without an anaesthetic, it should be a therapeutic premise to give the indicated dose of morphine sulphate by intramuscular injection 15 minutes (or by intravenous injection 5 minutes) before the procedure. There may be exceptions to this rule if the patient is already sedated, or there is some other contraindication to the drug, but it greatly reduces the pain and discomfort of what doctors are too often prepared to regard as a 'minor' procedure.

Preoperative Medication

General Anaesthetic

The anaesthetist will in most cases wish to prescribe the premedication himself. If not, the following is a useful guide. Premedication should be given from ¾ to 1 hour prior to operation. *N.B.* It is usually given by subcutaneous injection, but if there is any measure of peripheral vasoconstriction it *must* be given IM or IV

Under 3/12	Atropine 0.2 mg
3/12 to 1 year	Atropine 0.3 mg
1 to 2 years	Atropine 0.4 mg
2 to 10 years	Atropine 0.6 mg
10 to 15 years	{ Morphine 8 mg { Atropine 0.6 mg

15 to 60 years	{ Morphine 10 mg Atropine 0.6 mg
Over 60 years	{ Morphine 8–10 mg Atropine 0.6 mg

Morphine 10 mg approximately equals omnopon 20 mg.

Local Anaesthetic

A suggested scheme is (but individual preferences vary widely):

Triflupromazine	15 mg
Pethidine	100 mg

Adult: IM One hour preoperatively.
  Half this dose can be repeated IV immediately prior to operation if necessary, and further IV dosage may be used as required.
Child: Use a correspondingly smaller dose.

N.B. Occasionally severe falls of blood pressure occur especially if the patient sits up.

Postoperative Medication for Pain Relief and Sleep

Much can be done by counselling the patient upon what is to be expected. The house surgeon should keep his techniques simple. Some general points are:

For minor surgery *one* postoperative administration of an opiate is adequate and can be followed by minor analgesics such as pentazocine (Fortral) 30 mg IM or aspirin.

For major surgery or in situations where pain is severe (e.g. occasionally after haemorrhoidectomy) an opiate should be prescribed in regular doses so that pain is abolished. It is no use writing '4 hourly p.r.n.' for in this circumstance the drug will only be given if the patient complains. The instruction should read '*strictly* 4 (or 6) hourly'. Usually this is only required for 24 hours and may of course need modification to suit individual circumstances.

The following dosages are a useful guide. (Children frequently do not require post-operative opiates, but if necessary it is safe to give morphine in the dosages recommended.)

Under 10 years	Morphine 0.2 mg/kg up to 4 hourly

10–15 years	Morphine 8–10 mg up to 4 hourly
15 to 60 years or or	Morphine 10 mg Omnopon 20 mg Pethidine 100 mg up to 4 hourly
Over 60 years or	Morphine 8–10 mg Pethidine 50–100 mg up to 4 hourly

Increasing use is being made of continuous intravenous infusions of opiates to control initial severe post-operative pain. A motor driven syringe is best for this purpose and usually a rate of 2 mg morphine an hour suffices. When the patient has recovered from the general effects of anaesthesia and is beginning to experience pain, 15 mg of morphine sulphate is drawn up in 5–10 ml saline and administered at the rate of 1 ml every 15–30 seconds until pain is completely relieved and, in the case of an abdominal or thoracic operation, respiratory movements are completely free. This 'titration dose' is then used to determine the rate of delivery on the basis that the dose, divided by 6, is the hourly rate. If opiate drugs have been used for the anaesthetic and particularly if opiate reversal with nalorphine has been undertaken, great caution should be observed with this technique.

Other methods of pain relief are gaining popularity, particularly extradural administration of morphine or other opiates. You should be clear exactly what is to be done and by whom, and where to turn for advice.

In the relief of acute pain of known origin preoperatively, insufficient use is made of the same technique of taking 15 mg of morphine, diluting in 10 ml of saline and injecting this intravenously at a rate of 1 ml/30 sec until pain is relieved. Not only is this a very quick way of obtaining relief, but also a small total dose, 5–7 mg, is usually required.

The use of continuous intravenous morphine does carry a slight risk of overdosage characterised by a drowsy uncooperative patient, sometimes with a slow respiratory rate. This situation then joins the host of others that are responsible for mental confusion in the post-operative state. The diagnosis can be made and the situation reversed by the use of naloxone hydrochloride 400 micrograms intravenously, repeatedly if necessary. The patient will recover but the post-operative pain for which the morphine was given will also recur.

Do not forget that the patient needs sleep as well as relief from pain. Sleep rhythms are disturbed after surgery and help is often needed, particularly when the patient is trying to convalesce in an open ward. Barbiturates are rather out of fashion for this purpose, but if they are habitually being taken they are better continued. For the anxious patient, injectable diazepam 2–5 mg is sound. For those who can take drugs by mouth nitrazepam (5–10 mg) or dichloral-phenazone (Welldorm) 650 mg are usually satisfactory. Avoid ringing the changes on these or any other drugs of common properties such as antidepressants. The differences are usually small and their therapeutic efficacy is at least in part based on your understanding of the circumstances and your 'feel' of how they should be used. The latter can only be acquired if you stay with a small number of preparations.

The Lost Swab and the Wrong Operation

We will not deal with your many important duties while assisting in the operating theatre or carrying out operations yourself, except to draw your attention once again to certain real dangers:

1. The operation is performed on the *wrong patient*. In many hospitals all patients are labelled on admission: the name and hospital number on the label should be checked against the name and number appearing on the operating list. It is wise for you or the anaesthetist to undertake this check before induction of the anaesthetic, and/or to identify the patient by sight.

2. The operation is performed on the *wrong side* or on the *wrong digit*. Cases do occur of the wrong kidney, the wrong lung or the wrong limb being removed, or the wrong hernial orifice being explored. Sometimes this occurs because of incorrectly labelled X-rays, sometimes because of faulty memory on the part of the surgeon. It is wise to follow a regular routine of either *marking the side of operation* in the ward with indelible ink, or *confirming the affected side with the patient* before he is anaesthetised, or otherwise identifying the correct side. A special problem exists in the case of digits: it is wise to describe those of the upper limb by the old-fashioned terms of *thumb*, *forefinger*, *middle finger*, *ring finger* and *little finger*, rather than by numerals.

3. A *swab or instrument is left inside the patient*. This situation should first be recognised before the patient leaves the operating theatre. This can only be accomplished if a proper *count of swabs and instruments* is undertaken before and after the operation, and it is the surgeon's or your duty to *enquire specifically* from the scrub nurse whether the counts are correct. If no other written record is kept, write into the operation note 'Swabs and instruments correct'. All swabs are now marked with radio-opaque threads. If there is any anomaly in the count, the appropriate region of the patient should be *X-rayed* before he leaves the operating theatre table. It is of particular importance that no swabs or similar material or instruments are introduced into or taken from the theatre (e.g. with removed operative specimens) during the course of an operation.

A good account of the whole position in regard to this danger appears in the *British Medical Journal* of 26th January, 1963, and we suggest that you consult this as well as making yourself thoroughly acquainted with the rules for preventing loss of swabs and instruments laid down in your hospital.

Local Anaesthesia

1. *Lignocaine* is the standard local anaesthetic used.
2. *The maximum* 'safe' dose of this drug is about **0.5 g**

$$= 100 \text{ ml } 0.5\% \text{ solution}$$
$$= 25 \text{ ml } 2\% \text{ solution}$$

The 0.5% solution should be used for all common purposes other than special nerve blocks.

3. When *adrenaline* is included with the lignocaine solution, the concentration is such that the maximum 'safe' dose of adrenaline (0.5 ml 1/1000) will not be exceeded unless that of lignocaine is also. Adrenaline should *never* be used in a digital nerve block. Adrenaline should be used with caution in patients with some forms of heart disease.

4. If *overdosage* of lignocaine should occur (muscle twitching, convulsions):

Ensure airway, by intubation if necessary
Give oxygen
Give sod. thiopentone IV slowly till convulsions cease
Call an anaesthetist.

Minor Surgical Procedures

The houseman may frequently be called upon to undertake minor procedures such as superficial biopsy, liver biopsy, pleural and peritoneal paracentesis. This Guide is not a textbook on techniques and you must look elsewhere, particularly to your immediate seniors, for firm guidance. However, the following general points are applicable:

1. Always use adequate preliminary sedation. A small dose of morphine sulphate (5–10 mg) intravenously plus a little chlorpromazine (5–25 mg) detaches the patient from his environment and so makes you and him feel more at ease. Also, see page 20.

2. Infiltrate *widely* with dilute local anaesthetic (0.5 lignocaine).

3. For lymph node biopsy make an adequate incision (2 cm) so that you are not struggling for exposure or to control bleeding. If you make a good job of suture the scar will be invisible. Don't pull on the node—the pathologist will hate you!

4. For needle cutting biopsies such as breast, liver or prostate, make sure:
   (a) you understand the way the needle cutting combination works
   (b) you have incised the skin with a pointed scalpel
   (c) you are aware of the hazards (e.g. the need to keep the patient still during liver biopsy)
   (d) you have learnt the 'house rules' for the procedure.

5. If the lesion for biopsy appears to you to be doubtful (e.g. a possible malignant melanoma) don't do it—seek advice.

6. Don't hesitate to request technical help. Procedures may be thrown at you because you are thought to be competent. You lose nothing by admitting inexperience.

3. LABORATORY INVESTIGATIONS

General

There are three good and one bad reasons for doing investigations. The good are:

1. To enable a *decision* about diagnosis or management to be made.

2. To *screen* individuals at risk for particular conditions which may affect their management.

3. To establish a *baseline* against which change can be studied.

Examples of the first are liver function tests and ultrasound examination in the diagnosis of jaundice and a serum amylase investigation in a patient shortly after partial gastrectomy who collapses with acute abdominal pain.

Examples of the second are chest X-rays before surgery and electrocardiographic studies in patients with degenerative peripheral arterial disease.

Examples of the third are serum electrolyte concentrations in patients undergoing gastrointestinal surgery and preoperative laryngoscopy in thyroid surgery.

The bad reason is because you were told to do it in case it was 'wanted' or 'might prove useful'.

House surgeons are not always free agents but they should carry this classification in their mind and resist the temptation to do what are often unpleasant and costly things unless they fit into the framework of management.

Sources of Error

Although the results of these investigations are reported numerically, they are not necessarily more accurate than clinical findings in an individual case. That is, laboratory findings are subject to error.

The chief sources of error are:

1. *Sampling errors.* These apply to the collection of all specimens, and the source of error may be quite obscure unless specifically sought. So far as blood sampling is concerned, certain elementary precautions must be taken:

   (a) *Surgical spirit* (70%) only should be used as skin preparation. Small amounts of detergent entering the sample via the needle may result in significant haemolysis.
   (b) The plunger and barrel of the *syringe* must fit.
   (c) *Autoclaved*, *dry-heat sterilised* or *disposable* syringes should be used—never boiled ones.
   (d) *Dirty* (though sterile) syringes should be discarded.
   (e) A *tourniquet* may be used to locate the vein and for the

introduction of the needle. *Before* the blood sample is taken the tourniquet should be *released*, for venous congestion may lead to errors of up to 10% in for instance haematocrit and plasma protein.

(f) *Forearm exercise* before taking blood may lead to falsely high [K⁺] values.

(g) Blood should not be squirted through a fine needle into the sample bottle—this may cause *haemolysis*.

(h) For *blood gas estimations* to be of any value, the blood must at all times be protected from air. Blood (usually arterial) should be collected in a heparinized disposable syringe, the needle stopped with a cork, and immediately transported to the laboratory.

(i) *Speed* in the sample reaching the laboratory is of importance.

2. *Laboratory errors*. In general these are of two types:

(a) *Random*. These may be human or technical and occur with a frequency inversely proportional to the quality of the laboratory. Autoanalysers have greatly reduced the sources of random error, but no laboratory is yet entirely free of them.

(b) *Systematic*. These, too have been greatly reduced by means of autoanalysers, especially by their sophisticated inbuilt quality control systems, and by accompanying computer data-storage and retrieval systems that allow a much more exact determination of what range of values should be regarded as normal for a particular investigation, in a patient of a particular age and sex, in a particular hospital.

THE IMPORTANCE OF THESE SOURCES OF ERROR IS THAT A MAJOR DECISION WHICH DEPENDS ON A SINGLE LABORATORY RESULT, PARTICULARLY WHEN IT IS UNEXPECTED, SHOULD NEVER BE TAKEN WITHOUT REPEATING THE ESTIMATION.

3. *Errors of interpretation*. With increasing systematisation of sampling, automation of laboratory tests and the printout of their results, sampling and laboratory errors have been greatly reduced. However, automation has also brought with it a vastly greater capacity to generate laboratory data, and has accentuated another source of error: interpretation of data by the clinician. Instead of being presented with laboratory information bit by bit, he is now faced with large chunks, and for the most part finds difficulty in interpreting it in relation to the symptoms and signs that the par-

26

ticular patient exhibits. At the same time the clinician is faced with the enormous growth in quantity of other sorts of data, derived from radiologic, radionuclide, ultrasonic, thermographic, and similar tests, each with its own unique sources of technical and interpretive error. To these must be added the dimension of time, within which the patient, his disease, his doctor, and these numerical and graphical data vary.

There is little doubt that the solution to this new problem of information overload lies in the generator of the problem: the computer. Regrettably, computer-assisted medical decision-making is still in its infancy, and progress has lagged far behind the capacity to generate new data. But between this edition and next it can be anticipated that house surgeons will be gaining computer-assistance of this kind. (We said this in the last edition and we continue to live in hope).

Laboratory Nomenclature, and Metric (SI) Units

The house surgeon should be aware of the changes that are taking place in laboratory nomenclature, especially that used for enzymic estimations. Clinical biochemists, like most mortals, are finding it difficult to arrive at international agreement about the nomenclature and methods of estimating enzymic activity: as an Appendix we have listed some of the enzymic estimations in common use, and what has become the agreed nomenclature and abbreviations.

The house surgeon will also be aware that what he thought was the metric system has changed. In the Système Internationale (SI) there are no longer milliequivalents but millimoles; no longer mmHg but kilopascals; and so forth. Because of the confusion that necessarily accompanies change, we have included a further Appendix containing a tabular account of the SI system and the corresponding abbreviations.

Reference Values

'Normality' must refer to a sub-set of the population which is to be tested for 'abnormality'. Thus normal values determined, for instance, from a population of healthy medical students or nurses are quite meaningless if applied to an inpatient hospital population. Because of the not inconsiderable difficulty of defining a 'normal' inpatient, the term 'reference value' or 'reference range' is now often used.

In any biological system or population there is variance, so that no single numerical value can be referred to as an index of normality. In practice therefore laboratories provide a reference range of values, within which 90% or 95% of values obtained from the reference 'normal' population will lie. An abnormal value can be defined simply as one that lies outside this range. With more precision the degree of deviation from the reference range can be indicated on a percentile basis.

The reference range must incorporate not merely the biological variance in the population being tested, but also all sampling and laboratory errors which obtain in everyday practice. Quite evidently the methods of measurement used in a laboratory, and the units in which the results are expressed, will also affect the numerical values of reference ranges.

From the above it is clear that the reference ranges of laboratory values are unique to your own hospital laboratory and hospital population. In hospitals that use automated techniques laboratory results are printed out by computer, together with the reference range for the particular hospital population, and an index of the deviation of the individual results from the reference range. There is little purpose, therefore, in continuing to provide a table of 'normal' values within this text. As an appendix at the end, reference values from the Institute of Medical and Veterinary Science of South Australia are given, in order to give a general idea of normality.

Microbiology

Whenever an infection is detected in a patient a bacteriological sample must be sent for culture. This applies to throat swabs, sputum samples, swabs from wounds or boils, urine, blood culture. Antibiotic treatment should *never* start until this has been done.

Microbiological laboratories are usually fully staffed only in day-light hours. At other times, material may be taken with specially designed swabs which contain a nutrient medium, or may be plated out on agar plates which are obtained from a refrigerator and placed in an incubator. It is vital to ensure that a request form accompanies the specimen, and that there are reliable arrangements for it to reach the laboratory first thing the following morning.

28

It is increasingly being recognised that bacteroides organisms—normal inhabitants of the large bowel—play an important part in many surgical infections—e.g., acute appendicitis and after colon surgery. These organisms are facultative anaerobes and are not easily cultured unless

(a) the specimen goes straight into Stewart's transport medium

(b) anaerobic techniques are subsequently used.

Supplies of Stewart's medium should be kept available in and out of hours.

Where *bacteriological identification* may be *life-saving* or some unusual infection is suspected, the microbiologist on duty should be consulted.

Histology and Morbid Anatomy

Every operation specimen must be sent to the pathologist for histological examination. You must ask when *not* to obtain histology not the converse. When the result is required within 2–3 days the request form should be marked 'urgent'. *Frozen sections* are undertaken by special prearrangement. Some laboratories operate a 'rapid turnround' system by which a specimen delivered (say) by 9.30 a.m. is reported on by 4.30 p.m. This can be very useful in scheduling operations for breast lumps where preoperative diagnosis of cancer obtained by using a needle biopsy may make a frozen section unnecessary.

A frequent problem is that specimens are not sent to the pathologist in prime condition. There are usually local rules, but the following are always applicable:

1. Mucosal biopsies (e.g. from the colon or rectum) are pressed out onto a piece of thick card before being immersed in fixative. This helps the pathologist to orientate them and stops them curling up. Lymph node biopsies, especially where lymphomas are suspected, are best prepared by immediate imprint of the transversely cut surface on to a glass slide which is air dried. The cut node is then immersed in 10% formalin.

2. Organ specimens should be pinned out on cork. A salient point such as the apex of a dissection for cancer is identified by a marker—a black, silk stitch does very well—and this fact mentioned in the request form.

29

3. If a hollow viscus has not been emptied or opened consider whether you need to insert preservative into the lumen to ensure even fixation.

4. Whenever possible get round these problems by delivering specimens yourself.

Remember that you are obtaining an opinion from a consultant, and he cannot give help unless *full clinical details* including the existence of previous biopsies are supplied on the request form.

Haematology

Haematologic screening has now also become automated, mainly by way of cell counters and sizers, so that a much more comprehensive set of cell counts, sizes, types, and content is now available on a routine basis, often with a computer-printed diagnosis or suggestion for further investigation. Nevertheless, if the result seems unusual, or is not susceptible to full interpretation, do not hesitate to *consult with the haematologist*.

4. SPECIAL INVESTIGATIONS

Gastric Secretory Function Tests

There is little indication for these tests in the routine diagnosis of gastric or duodenal ulcer, but they may be of value in three circumstances:

1. In patients suspected of having the Zollinger–Ellison syndrome.

2. In the diagnosis of pernicious anaemia.

3. The investigation of patients with recurrent dyspepsia after surgical treatment.

These tests measure the amount of hydrochloric acid secreted, and the pH of the secretion, over a period of time or as a result of a stimulus. It is desirable to know the absolute quantity of acid secreted, which is the product of the concentration and volume. All depend on the proper placement of the gastric tube. Whenever possible a Salem double lumen tube size 14 or 16 French gauge should be inserted into the stomach so that free aspiration of gastric juice is obtained. For reliable results, the patient should be supervised throughout the test by a trained nurse or a doctor.

Maximum stimulation tests

The stomach can be made to secrete acid to its maximum by using either histamine or a synthetic gastrin (the penta-peptide pentagastrin). The latter is now used as it avoids the very slight possibility of reaction to histamine. The test gives a rough measure of parietal cell mass and is thus useful in determining if the patient is in the 'duodenal ulcer range' and possibly also in assessing patients after surgery.

All antacids and cimetidine should be withheld for at least 24 hours prior to the test. The patient is fasted for 12 hours and the gastric tube is inserted. *Basal secretion* is collected by continuous gastric aspiration for a period of 60 minutes. Thereafter pentagastrin 6 μg/kg IM is given and the gastric aspirate is collected every 15 minutes for a further 60 minutes. *The maximal acid output* is that quantity of acid contained in the two consecutive 15 minute collections which have the highest acid output. This result is multiplied by two. Typical results in mmol/hr of hydrochloric acid are shown in Table 1.

Table 1

normal		gastric ulcer		duodenal ulcer		pernicious anaemia	
BAO	MAO^{PG}	BAO	MAO^{PG}	BAO	MAO^{PG}	BAO	MAO^{PG}
Men							
2–4	25–45	0.5–3	15–35	3–6	30–60$^+$	0	0–0.25
Women							
1–3	20–40	0.5–2	10–25	3–5	25–50	0	0–0.25

BAO = Basal Acid Output
MAO^{PG} = Maximal Pentagastrin Stimulated Output

31

1) These are average values and figures outside these ranges have little diagnostic significance in individual patients.
2) In patients who hypersecrete acid, the Zollinger–Ellison Syndrome should be suspected if the basal acid output exceeds 50% of the maximal stimulated output.

Note: Though pentagastrin is given in a dose of 6 μg/kg body weight in patients before gastric surgery, after a vagotomy has been performed the dose is increased to 10 μg/kg.

Insulin test meal (modified Hollander)

The secretion of acid by the stomach in response to hypoglycaemia is dependent upon the presence of intact vagal fibres to the stomach. This is a test of the completeness of vagotomy, and when the test is positive in the early postoperative period the chances of the patient developing a recurrent ulcer are higher. It should not be performed in patients over 65 years of age or in those where there is a history of diabetes mellitus, epilepsy or cardiac irregularities. To be adequate the blood sugar must fall to 2.5 mmol/1.

The patient fasts for 12 hours. The gastric tube is inserted. The patient is warned of the unpleasant side-effects of the hypoglycaemia.

The stomach is aspirated every 15 minutes for 1 hour and the samples placed in separate test tubes—these are the control samples.

Soluble insulin is then given intravenously, 0.2 units/kg body weight, up to a maximum of 12 units.

The stomach is aspirated every 15 minutes for a further 2 hours and the samples placed in separate test tubes—these are the test samples.

Blood is taken for blood sugar estimations, 30 minutes and 45 minutes after the insulin is given.

The labelled sequence of control and test samples is sent to the laboratory with a request for the total amount of acid and the concentration of acid in each sample to be measured. The patient is given a glucose drink immediately the test is completed.

The Hollander criteria demand that given an adequate fall in blood glucose the test is positive (i.e. vagal fibres are intact) if any one 15 minute sample following insulin shows a rise greater than 20 mmol per litre. If no acid is present in the basal samples, as is sometimes the case after vagotomy, a rise of 10 mmol concentration is said to be positive. The test is unlikely to have any prognostic value when performed later than the first week after surgery.

Liver Function Tests

All jaundiced patients must have their status for hepatitis B determined and, until this is proved negative, special precautions in handling their blood are in order. In some units patients from high-risk areas (e.g. Africa, Middle East) are also screened.

Those most useful in surgical practice, and to be applied to every jaundiced patient, are:

> Serum bilirubin concentration
> Serum alkaline phosphate (ALP)
> Serum transaminase (AST)
> Serum albumin (and total protein)
> Prothrombin time or index

The most sensitive of the above tests to indicate hepatocellular damage is the AST level. While the concentration will steadily rise with increasing duration of bile duct obstruction, levels in excess of 500 i.u./l almost always indicate hepatitis and should be a warning against accepting a diagnosis of extrahepatic obstruction without other clearcut evidence. The above liver function tests, although sometimes providing a clearcut differentiation between a medical and surgical cause for jaundice, may be misleading as there is a substantial overlap between results for individual tests in various medical and surgical conditions. Another useful screening test is abdominal ultrasound which can, in many instances, provide confirmation of a diagnosis made on the basis of clinical examination and blood tests. (See the management of jaundice p. 150.)

Liver function tests have a wider role than merely investigating the patient who is presumed to have liver disease. They can *screen* for alcoholism when the glutamyl transferase is often raised; they are essential in the management of parenteral nutrition (p. 98); and the albumin level may be of use in nutritional deficiency, renal disease and in allowing standardisation of serum calcium concentration.

Cancer Antigens

Thus far, two proteins released into the blood stream by cancers, and detectable by immunologic means, have been recognised to have some diagnostic value. One is the *alpha-feto-protein* (or *-globulin*), which appears in the plasma in mg/ml quantities in about 85% of persons who develop hepatocellular carcinoma. The test has a low false-positive rate. Alpha-feto-protein may also be produced by malignant teratomas of the testis or ovary, when the plasma level may be of value in monitoring the response to therapy.

The other is the *carcinoembryonic antigen (CEA)* sometimes called the tumour-associated antigen (TAA), present in ng/ml amounts in patients with a variety of cancers: large bowel, pancreas, lung, breast and urinary tract in particular. It is also present in some patients with alcoholic cirrhosis, pancreatitis, and some apparently normal persons. Few laboratories have established proper tolerance limits for plasma CEA in non-cancerous patients. However, at best the clinical value of plasma CEA estimation as a diagnostic test for cancer is low, because a 70–80% false negative rate is necessary in order to achieve a false positive rate as low as 5%. In cancer patients with elevated levels at the time of initial diagnosis and treatment, serial CEA estimations have been used as a guide to persistence or recurrence of tumour.

A variety of other antigens (oncofetal and other), and other biochemical 'markers', have been proposed as indicating the presence of cancer but none is sufficiently discriminatory for clinical use.

Tests for Immune Status in Cancer

A number of tests of immune function have been proposed for cancer patients in general, or for those with certain specific cancers, with the purpose of providing guidance about prognosis or as to whether some form of immunotherapy might be of benefit. Apart from a general tendency for depressed cell-mediated immunity to be associated with a poor prognosis none has yet stood up to rigorous scrutiny as being useful in clinical practice.

Autoantibodies and other Antigens

Blood tests for a variety of other antigens and antibodies are now fairly freely available. In many cases their diagnostic value is not yet numerically defined, but a list is appended, together with conditions in which they may be positive:

34

Thyroid antibodies
  Thyroid microsomal   } Hashimoto's disease
  Thyroglobulin   } Primary myxoedema
  Thyroid stimulating
    immunoglobulin (TSIg)   Graves' disease

Gastric antibodies
  Parietal cell   }
  Intrinsic factor   } Pernicious anaemia

Adrenal antibodies   Idiopathic (non-tuberculous)
                           Addison's disease

Antibodies in liver disease
  Smooth muscle   Chronic active hepatitis
                           (if HBsAg negative)
  Mitochondrial   Primary biliary cirrhosis

Hepatitis antigens/antibodies
  Hepatitis B surface antigen
    (HBsAg)   Hepatitis B or carrier state
  Hepatitis B antibody   Indicative of past infection
    (anti HBs)   with HB virus
  Hepatitis B core antibody May indicate continuing viral
    (anti HB_c)   replication in the liver when
                         an isolated finding
  Hepatitis Be antigen and   Only in HBsAg positive sera,
    antibody   the former indicates high
    (HB_eAg and anti HB)   infectivity
  IgM antibody to hepatitis A Specific for recent infection
    virus   with HA virus

Reticulin antibodies   Coeliac disease, dermatitis
                           herpetiformis

Glomerular basement
  membrane antibodies   Goodpasture's syndrome

Skin intercellular antibody Pemphigus

Skin basement membrane
  antibody   Pemphigoid

Striated muscle antibodies

Acetylcholine esterase receptor antibodies	Myasthenia gravis
Rheumatoid factor(s)	Rheumatoid arthritis
Antinuclear antibodies	Various connective tissue diseases including SLE
Native DNA antibodies	Systemic lupus erythematosus (SLE)
Antibodies to extractable nuclear antigens (ENA)	Various connective tissue diseases, high titre anti-RNP antibody particularly characteristic of mixed connective tissue disease

Urinary Tract

Urine specimens

Male: The conventional mid-stream specimen is used.

Female: As a routine, the special clean mid-stream specimen is used. Only if there is any doubt about the result should resort be made to the catheter specimen.

The specimen should reach the laboratory within *one hour*. Out of hours, specimens will keep in the refrigerator (not the ice compartment!) overnight.

1. Microscopical examination for *pus cells* and *casts*. When chronic pyelonephritis is sought, a *quantitative white cell count* may be valuable—WBC excretion should be < 100 000/h; > 200 000/h is abnormal.

2. *Quantitative bacterial culture* and assessment of in vitro *antibiotic sensitivities*. Bacterial count should be < 10 000 organisms/ml.; > 100 000/ml is definitely abnormal, *provided* less than 1 hour has elapsed after voiding.

Bladder cytology

Cytological examination of the urine has proved of some value in the investigation of suspected bladder papilloma or carcinoma and the cytological appearance gives some indication of the degree of malignancy. Specimens should *not* be early morning ones. An equal volume of 10% formalin is added *at once*. Cytology is also useful in follow-up of patients with bladder cancer. For best results the voided urine should be collected directly into formalin to preserve cell morphology.

Creatinine clearance test

It is valuable when long term changes in renal function are to be sought.

1. Record *height* and *weight* on request form.
2. Fast from *meat*, *fish*, *tea* and *coffee* from 9 p.m. the previous night.
3. Patient must remain *in bed or at rest* during the test.
4. *Water load:* between 7 a.m. and 8 a.m. give 750 ml of fluid by mouth, and subsequently 100 ml/h for the duration of the test.
5. 8 a.m.: patient *empties bladder—discard urine.*
6. Collect *all urine* passed from 8 a.m. to 11 a.m. and send to laboratory.
7. Collect *all urine* passed between 11 a.m. and 2 p.m. and send to laboratory.
8. Collect *20 ml of blood* at 10 a.m. and send to laboratory.

Some units prefer, in some special circumstances, to extend the urine collection period over 24 hours.

Prostatic biopsy

This, by the transrectal or transperineal route, has replaced prostatic massage as the method of obtaining a diagnosis in prostatic cancer. It is usually done by an expert, but see Minor Surgical Procedures, p. 24.

Endoscopy

Attempts to examine hollow organs visually through a tube passed into them are of very considerable antiquity. Most were crude and ineffective until the development of small, low-temperature electric bulbs and more recently fiberoptics.

For successful endoscopy of any organ the three essential provisions are a source of light, a channel or optical arrangement to see through, and a translucent medium (gas or liquid) to separate the wall of the organ from the optical objective. The light source may introduce a burning or explosion hazard. The optical channel influences the size and flexibility of the instrument. The translucent medium may over-distend or even rupture the organ, or may enter veins or other undesirable sites. These necessities may also introduce difficulties in cleaning and sterilising the instruments.

The greatest advance in the last few years has been the conducting of light (illumination and images) through flexible bundles of fibres, referred to as the fiberoptic system. Although flexible, these systems are expensive, easily damaged, and are sometimes sterilised only with difficulty.

In Table 2 the characteristics of some of these instruments are summarised: their range, and their diagnostic and therapeutic applications. This is to indicate to you what useful information might be gained about your patient by endoscopic means. A brief description of each instrument, how it is used, and some of the hazards of its use are outlined below.

Proctoscopy

The proctoscope is a short, wide, open-ended tube through which the anal canal and lower few centimetres of the rectum can be examined. Built-in illumination is normally provided. No special preparation or anaesthesia is required. The knee-chest position is best, but the lateral position is more usual. A digital examination is made first and the patient then told to expect an instrument of approximately the same size. Do not proceed if the digital examination causes severe pain. The instrument with its obturator in place is warmed, lubricated, and gently introduced to its full length, pointing at the umbilicus. The obturator is then removed. First inspect the rectal mucosa for colour (salmon pink is normal), rugosity, ulceration, excess mucus and redundancy of folds. Then withdraw the instrument slowly, observing for piles and their prolapse through the sphincter. This investigation is well within the capacity of a house surgeon.

Sigmoidoscopy

Most diagnostic sigmoidoscopes are about 30 cm in length and up to 2 cm in diameter. They are hollow metal tubes with an obturator and a light source, which may be proximal, distal, or best of all fiberoptic. No special preparation of the patient is necessary or indeed desirable beyond possibly mild sedation. The left lateral position with the hips well flexed and raised on a pillow is best. The instrument should be warm, well lubricated and introduced to 5 cm pointing at the umbilicus. Then remove the obturator and advance the instrument under vision. In the lateral position a plain lens and air-insufflator are used to open up the lumen ahead of the instrument. If you encounter faeces, sneak the instrument alongside rather than trying to clean them out. Alternatively, give a disposable enema and repeat the examination. Considerable experience, skill, and care may be required to get round the rectosigmoid junction; in about half the patients this is impossible. Interpretation of what you see also requires considerable experience, but it is well within the capacity of a house surgeon to gain elementary skill with this instrument.

A flexible sigmoidoscope is now available and has greatly increased the range of examination. It is an instrument for the expert.

Colonoscopy

The colonoscope is a fiberoptic instrument and consequently flexible. Depending on the model, the skill of the operator, and the mobility of the colon it is possible to pass the instrument into the transverse colon and even the caecum. The instrument is now extensively used to diagnose inflammatory bowel disease and polyps.

Oesophagoscopy

The traditional oesophagoscope is a hollow brass tube illuminated by twin proximal lamps. Examination with this instrument is both difficult and dangerous, and should be left to your seniors. Although it is possible to carry it out under local anaesthesia, general anaesthesia is generally desirable. The danger arises from compression of the wall of the oesophagus between the instrument and the vertebrae, and from perforation of the oesophagus by the advancing tip. The advantage of this instrument is that foreign bodies can be

Table 2 Endoscopic procedures

Endoscope	Range of Instrument	Diagnostic Applications	Therapeutic Applications
Proctoscope	Anal canal Ano-rectal junction	Haemorrhoids, fissure, fistula, proctitis	Injection of haemorrhoids, Internal sphincterotomy
Sigmoidoscope	Rectum Lower ⅓ sigmoid	Diffuse mucosal changes (proctitis, colitis) Discrete lesions (polyp, cancer)	Removal of polyps Release of sigmoid volvulus Fulguration or cryo-destruction of cancer (palliative)
Colonoscope	Colon distal to splenic flexure Transverse and ascending colon	As above	Removal of polyps
Oesophagoscope	Oesophagus	Oesophagitis, stricture, cancer, foreign body	Dilation of stricture Removal of foreign body
Laparoscope	Liver, gallbladder, spleen Ovaries, tubes, rectovaginal pouch	Liver tumours, peritoneal metastases Pelvic inflammatory disease Ectopic pregnancy	Tubal destruction

Endoscope	Range of Instrument	Diagnostic Applications	Therapeutic Applications
Cystoscope	Bladder, bladder neck, urethra	Inflammation, tumour, stone, injury Retrograde urography	Fulguration tumour Extraction ureteric stone
Resectoscope	Bladder, bladder neck, posterior urethra	As above	Resection prostate, bladder neck, bladder tumour
Gastro-duodenoscope	Stomach (except close to cardia) All the duodenum	Diffuse mucosal changes (varices, gastritis, erosions, linitis plastica) Discrete lesions (ulcer, cancer, polyp)	Laser coagulation of bleeding vessels
Choledochoscope	Common bile and hepatic ducts	Exclusion of calculi	Nil
Bronchoscope	Down to orifices of 3rd order bronchi	Mucosal lesions (cancer) Compressive lesions (nodes) Origin of pus or blood	Bronchial toilet
Thoracoscope	Parietal, visceral pleura	Pleural lesions (cancer, tuberculosis, bullae)	Little used

removed, biopsies taken, dilatations, injections and other manipulations carried out in a way not easy with the fiberoptic oesophagoscope.

The fiberoptic oesophagoscope is much safer, and can be used under local anaesthesia. It allows an adequate view but less manipulation, though biopsies are easy.

Gastroduodenal endoscopy

Classical rigid and semi-rigid gastroscopes have been replaced by the flexible fiberoptic gastroscope. This can be passed under minimal sedation with local anaesthesia of the pharynx. The stomach has to be empty (or emptied), and is distended with air. It is possible to get a good view of the distal oesophagus, the whole of the stomach and the duodenum at least to its fourth part. Biopsies can be taken and a record made using a camera. The instrument is of great value in making the differential diagnosis between ulceration and cancer, and in identifying a source of bleeding. Interpretation of what is seen requires specialised skills.

Endoscopic retrograde pancreatico-duodenography (ERCP).

At duodenoscopy a catheter can be passed into the papilla and a retrograde injection made which outlines the biliary tree, the pancreatic duct, or both. Minor surgical procedures of slitting the papilla to release stones are possible. The investigation has an important role in the diagnosis of jaundice (p. 150) and abdominal pain thought to originate in the pancreas. Possible complications are chiefly the possibility of a raised serum amylase concentration—usually transient—after successful intubation of the pancreatic duct and ascending cholangitis; preventative chemotherapy should be discussed in the potentially septic case.

Choledochoscopy

The choledochoscope is introduced into the common bile duct at operation, and can be passed upwards at least to the junction of the right and left hepatic ducts, and downwards to the duodenum. In its modern, fiberoptic and flexible, form it has regained popularity for excluding common bile duct calculi after exploration.

Bronchoscopy

The bronchoscope is one of the older generations of endoscopes. It is a hollow, rigid, open-ended, metal tube without an obturator and with a light source. It can be passed under general or local anaesthesia. This is usually quite a safe examination, so long as adequate ventilation is maintained. All of the third-order individual bronchial orifices can usually be examined by means of telescopes with a variety of angle objectives. Foreign bodies can be removed and biopsies taken. Bronchoscopy has been widely employed in treating post-operative atelectasis, but alternative methods are now more commonly used. The use of the bronchoscope as a diagnostic instrument requires special training, but it is within the capacity of a house surgeon to use it for bronchial toilet. A venturi inflation device is essential for therapeutic bronchoscopy. Fiberoptic bronchoscopes are now widely used.

Thoracoscopy

A thoracoscope is introduced into the pleural cavity under local anaesthesia through the chest wall after a pneumothorax. It is rarely used nowadays.

Laparoscopy

This is now a popular and much used investigation in patients with abdominal pain or suspected malignancy. Its value lies in the ability to exclude pelvic causes for acute or chronic pain and in the detection of hepatic metastases. Sterilisation by fulguration or clipping of the Fallopian tubes is also possible.

Cystoscopy and urethroscopy

Modern fiberoptic cystoscopes allow the visualisation of both bladder and urethra. Resectoscopes are equipped with a cutting mechanism (usually diathermy) which allows resection of the prostate, bladder neck, or bladder tumours. Cystoscopy can be performed after instillation of lignocaine jelly into the urethra, but general or regional anaesthesia are preferable (and are essential if biopsies are to be taken or resection performed). A urine culture should always be made before instrumentation of the urethra: cystoscopy in the presence of urinary tract infection is a potent cause of septicaemia. The fluid used to distend the urethra and bladder must be sterile, clear, of low electrical conductivity, and at body temperature. For diagnostic cystoscopy water is satisfactory, but during resections the fluid may enter the blood stream via transected vessels: isotonic glycine solution is therefore often used.

Many types of cystoscope are available and many accessories. You must warn the theatre staff of any procedures contemplated, such as ureteric catheterisation (single or double), fulguration, biopsy, etc., and of any special angles of view desired, so that correct telescopes are available.

Gentleness and skill in passing the instrument are important in avoiding injury to the delicate urethra, and to obtain a full view of the undisturbed bladder wall. Antibiotic cover is only used if there is clinical evidence of infection.

In middle-aged and elderly males cystoscopy may induce acute retention of urine, and these patients should always be admitted to hospital, if only as day patients.

Respiratory Function Studies in Relation to Surgery

Mention has already been made of the need for preoperative respiratory function studies in patients who may have respiratory 'problems'. These may be defined as:

1. Past history or present evidence of respiratory disease particularly chronic bronchitis or asthma.

2. Current cough or sputum or evidence that this occurs in unfavourable circumstances (e.g. winter).

3. Physical condition of the chest wall which may produce a restrictive defect.

In all these circumstances and in particular in the anticipation of major abdominal or thoracic surgery it is necessary to know three things

1. Is the vital capacity greater than three times the tidal air? If it is not then respiratory insufficiency is almost inevitable after a laparotomy or thoracotomy, the muscular disorganisation and pain of which are sufficient to reduce VC by about two thirds. With

appropriate action by the anaesthetist and the relief of pain (for example by epidural anaesthesia or continuous low dose intravenous morphine, p. 21) such patients need not go into respiratory failure but this is only true if all are prepared by appropriate information.

2. Is there an element of bronchospasm? This can be ascertained by comparing a low FEV_1 before and after the administration of bronchodilators such as an isoprenaline spray or a salbutamol inhaler. The presence of bronchospasm is an indication of likely postoperative trouble from sputum retention and calls for postponement of the operation until control of the situation can be achieved.

3. Is there a restriction on free chest movement? A patient's FEV_1 may be low in the absence of airways obstruction if the lung and/or the chest wall are stiff. Such patients faced with additional burdens in the postoperative period may develop respiratory failure or, just as important, may get fatigued. Again appropriate avoiding action can be taken if the risk is understood.

In addition to the above measurements, arterial blood gas tensions (pO_2, pCO_2,) should be determined as base-lines in all patients with a hint of respiratory disease who are to undergo major surgery. (See p. 104 for interpretations.)

5. RADIOLOGY AND OTHER IMAGING INVESTIGATIONS

The house-surgeon whose patient may need some form of organ imaging will make a request for the procedure and provide liaison between his clinical team and the imaging department. Such examinations must not be requested without good reason and only after full clinical examination. You must learn what imaging can and cannot reveal in different situations, and also which examinations you can request personally and which need to be authorised by a more senior doctor. In any event you must remember that the request is one for consultation with a very senior colleague and NOT an order for an examination. If unsure of the best approach to a problem, ask a consultant in imaging. If you go to the department to find out the result from the consultant, you will avoid delays, have firsthand knowledge and be able to carry out effectively your function of liaison.

While plain and contrast radiography (still, cine or videotape) remains the most common method of displaying normal or abnormal internal organs, and the chest film is still the most common request in a general hospital, considerable progress has occurred in other imaging methods, especially in computerised tomography (CT), ultrasound, and gamma imaging (radionuclide imaging, nuclear scanning, scintigraphy). The high cost of these techniques, and the relatively high radiation dose in CT and gamma imaging, must be weighed against greater diagnostic accuracy.

Costs vary from hospital to hospital. The following costs, expressed relative to the hospital bed cost per day, may serve as an approximate example:

	$A	£stg
Hospital bed cost per day	200	80–110
X-ray extremity, chest, spinal region, skull	30	12
Barium study, urogram, ultrasound, scintigram	40–80	30
Head CT scan	180	100
Body CT scan	230	240
Arteriogram, lymphangiogram, cerebral air study	200–300	200

Rapid advances in equipment and techniques are being made, and you will find it valuable to talk to the imaging consultant about any unusual problems. In all cases it is essential to give a full clinical summary on the request form to enable the imaging consultant to select the appropriate technique and to give the most helpful opinion.

Hazards

Because of their ionising effects, X-rays are dangerous. They increase the individual's chance of malignant disease and may also affect genetic tissue in ovary or testis. In consequence:

All X-rays should be kept to a minimum.

For females in the childbearing age the '10 day rule' should be applied when the examination is not truly urgent. Effectively this means five days before and five days after the midpoint of the menstrual cycle. Most X-ray Departments now specify this on their request forms.

In males, gonads should be protected where possible.

Plain Radiography

In order to save both you and the X-ray department time and trouble, the correct forms of request for certain common views are as follows:

Skull

PA, appropriate lateral and Towne's views.

Facial bones

Do not merely ask for 'X-ray facial bones', but ask for views of the bone thought to be fractured, e.g. malar views, maxillary views.

Cervical spine

AP, lateral, odontoid view, obliques.

Chest X-ray

PA chest, or in the case of portable X-ray, AP. Lateral views should be requested on initial examination. Erect views are most satisfactory but, if not possible, sitting views are usually more satisfactory than supine.

Ribs and sternum

The diagnosis of fractured rib or sternum is clinical and attempts to X-ray the fracture are of little value. A PA chest is usually necessary to detect lung damage and pleural abnormalities.

Abdomen

AP view, supine and erect if bowel abnormality is suspected. A 'lateral decubitus' view may be valuable, especially in patients too ill to stand. A lateral view may show an aortic aneurysm.

Thoracic and lumbar spine

PA and lateral views. Oblique or coned view may be required.

Pelvis and hips

AP view is sufficient as a preliminary in trauma. Lateral views may be required to confirm fracture, or in cases such as suspected slipped femoral epiphysis.

Mammography

This special technique of soft tissue radiography of the breast for cancer can be used with conventional X-ray film or by the special technique of xeroradiography. It is not a routine investigation; the radiation dose is too high for safe use in large scale cancer detection programmes, and special skills in interpretation are necessary. The main indications are as an aid to decision in some clinically benign or doubtful breast lumps, and as a screening technique in patients with a high risk of breast cancer (bad family history, cancer of other breast).

Contrast Radiography

Barium meal

This involves a study of the oesophagus, stomach and duodenum. If abnormality in the oesophagus or swallowing mechanism is suspected, this should be indicated on the request.

Barium meal and follow-through

This request is of little value unless the portion of the gastrointestinal tract to be examined is mentioned, e.g. the request might read 'barium meal and follow-through study of terminal ileum'. Barium meal or follow-through should *not* be requested in cases of suspected *intestinal obstruction*; a gastrografin meal may sometimes be useful and is safe.

Barium enema

Digital examination of the rectum must, and in general sigmoidoscopy should, be performed before a barium enema examination. However, a recent sigmoidoscopic biopsy is a contraindication to barium enema examination. It is a safe procedure in the presence of suspected or actual large bowel obstructions—oral barium studies are not.

Intravenous urography (pyelography)

This study still remains the best starting point for detecting abnormalities of the urinary system. In certain circumstances, such as in uraemia and multiple myeloma, dehydration should be avoided. Valuable information can be obtained even when the blood urea concentration is markedly raised, but it is essential that contact is made with the radiologist to discuss each case.

Retrograde urography (pyelography)

This study is of particular value in the investigation of obstructed or poorly functioning kidneys. As it needs the cooperation of a radiographer, the radiology department needs to be notified in advance to prevent unnecessary delays in theatre.

Voiding cystography and urethrography

Direct cystourethrography is of special value when injury to the urethra or bladder is suspected, as in fractured pelvis. However, never pass a catheter in suspected rupture of the urethra without the consent of the surgeon in charge. The house surgeon may be required to make the urethral injection of contrast (via a urethral nozzle), followed by injection into the bladder (by way of a gently introduced, soft, blunt-tipped catheter). If possible the study should be carried out under image intensification control to minimise extravasation.

Dynamic urography–urodynamics

Cine cystography and urodynamics (bladder and bladder neck dysfunction, vesico-ureteric reflux) should be arranged only after collaboration and consultation with radiologists and urologists.

Radiological investigation of the biliary tree

There are many methods for investigating the extrahepatic biliary tree, and the choice between ultrasound, gamma imaging and contrast radiography may be difficult. The various forms of cholegraphy are listed here; their place and management will be found under the headings of individual disorders.

Oral cholecystography is principally designed to examine the anatomy of the gallbladder, to detect calculi, and to assess its ability to concentrate and to contract. It is of no value in a jaundiced patient, and is usually not performed less than three weeks after an attack of biliary colic or cholecystitis if it is hoped positively to identify gallstones.

Intravenous cholangiography is used to demonstrate the major bile ducts, and sometimes the gallbladder. Because of the higher incidence of contrast reactions, it is usually replaced by ultrasound and percutaneous transhepatic cholangiography, or endoscopic retrograde bile duct cannulation (ERCP).

Percutaneous transhepatic cholangiography. The 'skinny' or Chiba needle is used to enter the bile ducts, allow bile aspiration, and to introduce contrast, particularly following ultrasound demonstration of dilated bile ducts. It is complementary to ERCP (p. 42) and is used to show the site and cause of obstruction. Coagulation defects should be tested for and if necessary Vitamin K given. Antibiotic cover is often indicated.

Operative cholegraphy. Many surgeons regard operative cholegraphy in patients with biliary tract disease as routine, as it may show unsuspected calculi and abnormalities of the biliary system. More important, it reduces the number of unnecessary duct explorations. Booking with the X-ray department is required.

Postoperative choledochography. When the common bile duct has been opened and a T-tube inserted, a choledochogram via the T-tube is requested for the 8–10th postoperative day to detect any residual calculi or obstruction. The T-tube must not be removed until this film has been inspected.

Arteriography. This is an invasive procedure with significant risks. In many cases discussion with the radiologist should occur before booking and examination. Clinical details should include the site and the nature of the lesion which is suspected and the route suggested for injection of the contrast, e.g. via right femoral artery, translumbar aortogram, etc. Apart from its use in the diagnosis of arterial disease, selective arteriography is used in the diagnosis or characterisation of tumours (e.g. kidney, liver, limb, brain) and to identify major bleeding sites in the GI tract (oesophageal varices, peptic ulcer, colonic diverticular disease).

There has been much progress in invasive angiography in recent years, and both embolisation via a catheter for bleeding sites, e.g. oesophageal varices and colonic diverticula, and preoperative embolisation of tumors, e.g. renal cell carcinoma, can be performed. Transluminal dilatation of atherosclerotic vessels particularly in the limbs is being assessed for long term results.

There is promise that a much less invasive form of arteriography will be available in future, in which the contrast medium is injected intravenously and the arteries delineated as it passes through them by means of a computerised subtraction technique: intravenous angiography.

Phlebography

Lower limb phlebography is the most accurate mode of diagnosing deep venous thrombosis. Selective retrograde phlebography is used in special circumstances e.g. renal, adrenal veins.

Lymphangiography

This is occasionally useful in staging and followup of lymphoma, where the CT scan is negative, but is more useful in the detection of pelvic metastases, e.g. carcinoma of the cervix. It is tedious to perform, especially in lymphoedema, when the results are seldom helpful.

Specialised Imaging Techniques—Ultrasound, CT and Gamma-Imaging

These techniques are in no way mutually exclusive, but rather are

51

Table 3 Common gamma-imaging procedures

Tissue region or organ	Radiopharmaceutical	Principle of uptake	Lesions revealed	Diagnostic accuracy
Lung (perfusion)	99mTc MAA	Embolisation of pulmonary capillaries	Pulmonary emboli	Excellent for large emboli. Fair for multiple small emboli.
Lung (ventilation)	133Xe	Inhaled diffusible gas	Uneven ventilation	Aids discrimination of pulmonary emboli from lung disease
Liver	99mTc phytate	Taken up by macrophages	Primary or metastatic tumours and cysts; extrinsic lesions invading or indenting liver	Good if lesions greater than 2 cm diameter
Spleen	99mTc phytate	Taken up by macrophages	Estimate of spleen size; ruptured spleen	Excellent
Gallbladder and ducts	99mTc PG	Taken up and excreted by hepatocytes	Obstruction of cystic or main bile ducts	Excellent

Tissue region or organ	Radiopharmaceutical	Principle of uptake	Lesions revealed	Diagnostic accuracy
Kidney	99mTc HIDA 99mTc DTPA	Excreted through glomeruli	Avascularity; space occupying lesion; obstructive uropathy; renal function residual urine volume; ureteric reflux	Fair to good
Other abdominal organs	99mTc O$_4$	Taken up by parietal cells	Meckel's diverticulum	Good
	67Ga citrate	Transferrin transport	Intra-abdominal abscess	Good
Thyroid	99mTc O$_4$ or 131I Na	Taken up by acinar cells	Region of avid uptake (toxic nodule, adenoma) Region of low or zero uptake (cancer, cyst)	Good
Bone	99mTc MDP	Taken up by osteoblasts	Primary or metastatic tumour; osteomyelitis; avascular necrosis	Excellent
Brain	99mTc DTPA	Normally does not cross blood-brain barrier	Region of abnormal vascularity eg tumour	Good
CSF shunt	99mTc O$_4$	Injected into shunt	Patency of ventriculo-atrial or peritoneal shunt	Excellent

Tissue region or organ	Radiopharmaceutical	Principle of uptake	Lesions revealed	Diagnostic accuracy
Heart	^{99m}Tc TSPP	Taken up by infarct	Myocardial infarct	Good after 3–5 days
	^{99m}Tc red cells	Blood pool	Dynamic studies of ventricular form and function	Good
	^{201}Tl Cl	K$^+$ analogue; incorporated into myocardium after exercise	Ischaemic heart disease	Good

Co = cobalt Cr = chromium Ga = gallium I = iodine Tc = technetium Tl = thallium Xe = xenon
DTPA = diethylene trianine pentacetic acid MAA = macro-aggregated albumin
MDP = methylene diphosphonate PG = pyridoxylidene glutamate HIDA = sodium N-diethylphenyl carbamoylmethyl iminodiacetate TSPP = tetra sodium polyphosphate

complementary, and the choice of studies should be made in each individual case. However, several guidelines can be laid down; for example, for anatomical and technical reasons, ultrasound is more useful in thin patients whereas CT is best used in obese patients. Gamma imaging demonstrates dynamic physiology, while both CT and ultrasound demonstrate static anatomical lesions. For example, biliary anatomy can be imaged by ultrasound, physiological function by gamma imaging and in certain circumstances both may replace contrast radiography (oral cholecystography).

The major advantage of ultrasound is the absence of ionising radiation, and it is thus considered safe for young patients and the foetus. Repeated and prolonged studies can also be performed, such as followup examinations during pregnancy, or prolonged biopsy procedures.

Ultrasound

High frequency ultrasound (2–10 MHz) is reflected from interfaces in body tissue, and converted to an image in shades of grey on a video monitor. The images are stored on videotape, paper or X-ray film. Manual contact scanning is most commonly used, but automated imaging (Octoson) and realtime scanning are also useful, and the images are now comparable to CT scanning, and therefore more readily acceptable to clinicians. It has an established place in obstetrics, neonatal paediatrics (placental site, foetal position, foetal abnormalities, multiple pregnancy) and cardiology. It is of value in making some diagnoses in general surgery: solid tumour versus cyst (thyroid, kidney), size of abdominal aortic aneurysm, presence of biliary tract obstruction. It is particularly useful for ultrasound guided biopsy, either tissue core or aspiration biopsy.

CT

Using a rapidly rotating scanning technique and finely collimated beams of X-rays, an image in shades of grey is built up and viewed on video screens, or X-ray films. It has an established place in neuroradiology, in which it has been largely able to replace invasive techniques such as ventriculography and cerebral angiography. In

Table 4, Guide to choice of method of imaging: CT scan ultrasound gamma-imaging

Organ, region or anatomical structure	Preferred technique
Intracranial contents	C.T. for anatomical abnormalities Gamma-imaging for blood flow
Thyroid	Ultrasound for solid vs cystic tumours, ultrasound for biopsy C.T. for staging of tumour Gamma-imaging for function
Mediastinum	C.T.
Heart	Realtime and M mode ultrasound for valve and ventricular function Gamma-imaging for function, infarct, ischaemia
Lungs	Gamma-imaging for respiratory function, pulmonary embolism C.T. for metastases and radiotherapy planning
Liver	Gamma-imaging, ultrasound, CT for metastases.
Biliary Tree	Gamma-imaging, ultrasound
Spleen	Gamma-imaging
Pancreas	C.T. for mass lesion, ultrasound for biopsy
Adrenal	C.T.
Kidney	Ultrasound for cyst vs tumour and aspiration or biopsy C.T. for staging tumour
Retroperitoneum (lymph nodes)	Ultrasound or C.T.
Aorta	C.T. for assessment of aneurysm prior to surgery, ultrasound for diagnosis, and follow up

Organ, region or anatomical structure	Preferred technique
Uterus and contents	Ultrasound for obstetrics and aspiration biopsy including amniocentesis
Pelvic organs	Ultrasound for ovary, C.T. for bladder, cervix, bowel tumour spread
Bone	Gamma-imaging

Consultation with the imaging consultant will provide further information on these and other procedures available, and may enable the procedure to be altered to solve the particular clinical problem presented.

---

the ten years since initial development of the CT scanner, assessment of its use in the chest and abdomen, as well as in the extremities, has established definite indications.

Gamma-imaging

The imaging device used is generally a gamma camera with quantification of data by computer processing where possible. The source of the image is a gamma-emitting, radionuclide-labelled compound or radio pharmaceutical which, because of either its physical or chemical properties, is organ specific.

Tables 3 and 4 indicate the organs commonly imaged, the radiopharmaceuticals used, the diseases commonly diagnosed, and a crude estimate of test accuracy.

6. ANTIBIOTICS AND CHEMOTHERAPY

Antibacterial drugs have undoubtedly contributed to reduced morbidity and mortality in modern surgery. There is however clear evidence that they are still widely misused in all hospital services, including surgery.

Probably the commonest identifiable area of misuse over the years has been in surgical prophylaxis and this continues. Many studies are now available which suggest how we might begin to use them more sensibly in this situation. It is also worth being reminded that no antibacterial drug is entirely free from side-effects and occasional lethal toxicity.

Some General Considerations

1. Where it is feasible, obtain appropriate specimens before starting antibacterial drugs.

2. Remember an urgent Gram stain of infected material may sometimes provide information rapidly which helps initial antibacterial selection.

3. Prescribe short courses of antibacterial drugs with a defined end-point.

4. Most abscesses need surgical drainage sooner rather than later: many surgeons will use antibacterials as well if there is a great deal of surrounding cellulitis. There is also evidence that a single pre-operative dose of rationally selected antibacterial diminishes operative bacteraemia at abscess drainage but no evidence that continuing antibiotics is useful.

5. Enquire about allergy critically and while it is legally safe to err on the cautious side, 'second line' alternative drugs are usually second line for a good reason. Much alleged 'allergy' is side-effects, e.g. diarrhoea and nausea.

6. Antibacterial selection in the first instance requires a knowledge of the likely causative organisms associated with particular clinical situations. It is impossible to use them sensibly without this basic knowledge.

7. Newer drugs generally cost more and are not necessarily better.

8. If in doubt ask for advice, no one knows everything.

Antibacterial Drugs

Penicillins

A large drug family with generally low toxicity. There is an enormous theoretical knowledge and practical experience with their use.

Benzylpenicillin (penicillin G, crystalline penicillin). This was the

58

original penicillin first used clinically in 1941. Still one of the treatments of choice for many infections, e.g. streptococcal cellulitis and impetigo, gonorrhoea, penicillin sensitive staphylococcal infections, pneumococcal pneumonia (the commonest cause of lobar pneumonia) and alone or as a component of regimens for less common surgical infections such as anaerobic chest disease, clostridial myonecrosis (gas gangrene) and other varieties of clostridial and anaerobic streptococcal cellulitis, tetanus, postoperative synergistic gangrenes (rare) and actinomycosis.

Only used parenterally with adult doses 2.0–12.0 (usually 2.0–6.0) Mu/day (depending on the particular clinical syndrome) given 2–6 hourly. Generally only used IV, though if needed IM, 1% lignocaine added reduces local pain.

Procaine penicillin. Only given IM. It provides a longer duration of penicillin activity for up to 24 hours. Used as a component of some regimens for gonorrhoea and syphilis and occasionally for patients with penicillin sensitive infections for whom low concentrations are acceptable, e.g. pneumococcal pneumonia.

Benzathine penicillin. Only given IM. It provides a very prolonged duration of low level penicillin action for about three weeks. Given monthly it is the most effective prophylactic regimen for preventing rheumatic fever, but has no surgical uses.

Penicillin V (phenoxymethylpenicillin). Only used orally where a patient has a penicillin sensitive infection and may reliably be expected to absorb the drug; e.g. streptococcal pharyngitis, impetigo and pneumococcal pneumonia. It is *not* effective as treatment for gonorrhoea or syphilis, and food markedly impairs its absorption.

Isoxazolyl penicillins (viz. cloxacillin, flucloxacillin and their relatives). These drugs are not significantly broken down by the beta-lactamase enzymes of *S. aureus* which confer penicillin resistance. Still considered the drugs of choice for all penicillin resistant staphylococcal disease. In most places upward of 75% of *S. aureus* both in and out of hospital are now resistant to benzylpenicillin. *S. pyogenes* are always sensitive to these drugs too. Cloxacillin may be given parenterally or orally, flucloxacillin only orally. Blood levels of flucloxacillin are about twice those of equal weight doses of cloxacillin. Dosage regimens are 1.0 g–12.0 g/day of cloxacillin (usually 1.0 g–4.0 g) given 4–6 hourly. Flucloxacillin dosage is 750 mg– 3.0 g/day given 6–8 hourly. Food impairs the absorption of both these drugs.

'Gram-negative' or 'broad spectrum' penicillins

Ampicillin. This drug added significant numbers of gram negative organisms, in particular *E. coli* and *Haemophilus influenzae*, to the spectrum of benzylpenicillin. It is used orally and parenterally. With the passage of time increasing resistance has developed amongst these organisms, e.g. up to 50% of *E. coli* may now be resistant; up to 10% of *H. influenzae* and up to 30% of *N. gonorrhoea*, although geographical variations are enormous and local information is important. The resistance of *E. coli* has unfortunately diminished the previously very useful role of ampicillin played in urinary tract infections and surgical abdominal sepsis. Adult dosage is 1.0–12.0 (usually 1.0–4.0) g/day given 4–6 hourly.

Amoxycillin. This drug has an identical microbiological spectrum to ampicillin which includes all benzylpenicillin sensitive organisms, many gram-negative bacilli and all enterococci. It is only used orally and results in blood levels twice those of ampicillin for the same weight dose; 500 mg ampicillin q.i.d. is equatable with 250 mg amoxycillin t.d.s. Amoxycillin's absorption is little affected by food.

These two drugs are still the most commonly prescribed antibiotics both in and out of hospital. Despite the trends in resistance mentioned, they remain useful for acute purulent exacerbations of chronic respiratory disease, acute otitis media, acute sinusitis, broncho-pneumonia, gonorrhoea (though complex resistance is emerging) acute pelvic inflammatory disease and urinary tract infection (if the bacteria are sensitive). Though diarrhoea and rash in particular may be troublesome, their widespread and continuing use reflects their low toxicity and high efficacy. In seriously ill patients, however, who may have septicaemia and for whom correct antibacterial selection is critical, they no longer provide adequate gram-negative bacillary cover. It is important to appreciate this.

Carbenicillin and ticarcillin. These drugs are used less frequently.

They add *Pseudomonas aeruginosa* in particular to the spectrum of ampicillin, although overall gram negative activity is better than ampicillin. Usually only used for proven or strongly suspected pseudomonas disease. Both are only given IV: Carbenicillin 20–30 g/day, ticarcillin 12–18 g/day. Both have high Na^+ concentrations (viz. 5 mmol/g of drug) which is potentially important in some patients with fluid and electrolyte imbalance. They can also cause hypokalemia and platelet dysfunction. The most costly antibiotics at present available, on a daily cost basis.

Cephalosporins

A family of broad spectrum bactericidal drugs, chemically related to penicillins. As a result of major pharmacological manipulation to increase their spectrum of gram negative activity, they are being used more frequently than previously in sick surgical patients. Cephalosporins have three generations which reflects their historical development and their increasingly broad spectrum of gram negative bacillary activity (see Table 5).

Table 5, Cephalosporins

First generation	Second generation	Third generation
Cephaloridine	Cefuroxime	Cefoperazone
Cephalothin	Cefamandole	Cefotaxime
Cephalexin*	Cefoxitin	Moxalactam
Cefazolin	Cefaclor*	
Cephradine*		

* Oral preparations. Only cephradine has parenteral preparations as well.

First generation drugs (cephalothin being the most familiar) have broad spectrum gram positive and negative activity. They act on penicillin sensitive and resistant (betalactamase producing) *S. aureus*, streptococci (not enterococci) and many gram negative

61

bacilli, e.g. many *E. coli*, and *Proteus mirabilis* in particular. In most places gram negative bacilli, including *E. coli*, have recently tended to develop increasing resistance to these drugs. It is this microbiological event which has stimulated the development of second and third generation cephalosporins resistant to the enzymes which break down their first generation relatives. Local resistance patterns of gram negative organisms should be known before deciding whether any of these cephalosporins, or which of them, might reasonably be used for gram negative bacillary disease. Cephalothin dosage is 1.0–8.0 (usually 1.0–4.0) g/day given IV 4–6 hourly.

Cefazolin can be given IM with less pain, and 8 hourly, which some regard as advantageous. Few important gram negative organisms are resistant to the second generation drugs, though how long this state of affairs will last remains to be seen.

Cefuroxime is conveniently administered as 0.75 g 8 hourly IV, and cefamandole as 1.0 g 4–6 hourly IV. Cefoxitin, alone of all cephalosporins so far, has significant activity against *Bacteroides fragilis*, the commonest anaerobic isolate in surgical abdominal sepsis. This property, allied to its broad spectrum aerobic gram negative bacillary activity, makes it satisfactory used alone for surgical abdominal sepsis in a dose of 1.0–2.0 g 6–8 hourly IV. However, it is the most expensive of a generally expensive family of drugs.

The third generation cephalosporins add activity against *Pseudomonas aeruginosa* to the spectrum of second generation drugs. They are at present still under trial.

Cephalosporins are relatively non-toxic; cephalothin increases the nephrotoxicity of aminoglycosides. Most need dosage reduction only with severe renal impairment but cephaloridine, the first cephalosporin, is in a separate category and is totally contraindicated in renal impairment. The combination of a cephalosporin and a loop diuretic (e.g. frusemide) is nephrotoxic. Allergy, diarrhoea and candidiasis may interfere with therapy. Cephalosporins are frequently recommended as alternative therapies for penicillin allergic patients unless there is a history of anaphylaxis or rapid onset hypersensitivity.

Aminoglycosides

Gentamicin and tobramycin are broad spectrum drugs (but with no activity against anaerobic organisms or streptococci). For over a decade they have been the mainstay of therapy in seriously ill patients with actual or presumptive gram negative bacillary sepsis. Nearly all important gram negative bacilli (*E. coli*, *Proteus* sp., *Klebsiella* sp., and *Ps aeruginosa*) remain sensitive. The well known problems of oto- and nephro-toxicity are minimised by measuring trough levels of drug and altering dosage and frequency if this rises above 2 mg/L ($=\mu$/ml). Careful adjustment of dose is needed in the presence of impaired renal function. Usual dosage is a loading dose of 2 mg/kg and then 5 mg/kg/day given 8 hourly with monitoring of the drug level.

The earlier aminoglycosides (e.g. streptomycin) are rarely used now. Amikacin is a derivative of the earlier kanamycin and is the most resistant member of this family to the aminoglycoside inactivating enzymes of gram negative bacilli. It is currently not for widespread use.

The nephrotoxicity of these drugs is undoubtedly enhanced by the concomitant administration of cephalothin. Caution should be observed and there can rarely be an indication to combine cephalosporins and aminoglycosides.

Metronidazole (and tinidazole)

Metronidazole has an extremely broad spectrum for anaerobes, but has no activity against aerobic or microaerophilic organisms. Virtually all *B. fragilis* isolates are sensitive to it. It is now widely used in many parts of the world alone or as a component of regimens for the management of abdominal sepsis, or prophylactically in large bowel surgery. Parenteral dosage is 500 mg 8–12 hourly IV (the latter dose is most often adequate) and is expensive. It is well absorbed orally (400 mg t.d.s. for anaerobic disease) and rectally as suppositories (0.5–1.0 g 8 hourly). Most patients who need the drug can receive it in either of these non-parenteral ways effectively and relatively cheaply. It is also effective against protozoa, e.g. *Entamoeba histolytica*, *Giardia lamblia* and *Trichomonas vaginalis*.

Tinidazole is a slightly less nauseating relative which can only be used orally. Its antimicrobial spectrum is identical. Both may give rise to a metallic taste in the mouth and be associated with a 'disulfiram reaction' with alcohol.

Sulphonamides

These were the earliest, widely and successfully used antibacterial

63

drugs but the development of resistance by many organisms reduced their usefulness. *E. coli*, the commonest cause of urinary tract infections, has in many places shown a tendency towards increasing sensitivity over recent years, perhaps related to their less frequent use. They are thus still often inexpensive and effective alternatives for urinary tract infections in particular. There are no clinically important differences between them and sulphadimidine is an effective simple sulphonamide to be arbitrarily selected.

Cotrimoxazole

This drug is a fixed combination of sulphamethoxazole and trimethoprim with broad spectrum gram positive and negative activity. It is mostly used for acute purulent exacerbations of chronic respiratory disease and for urinary tract infections. Diarrhoea is a not uncommon side-effect and severe skin rashes, ascribed to the sulphonamide component, are seen occasionally. Generally it is used on a 2 tablet (480 mg) b.d. dosage regimen but a parenteral preparation is available which contains large quantities of sodium. There is microbiological and clinical debate about the need for both drugs in this fixed combination and moves are afoot in some parts of the world to use trimethoprim alone.

Chloramphenicol

This is a famous, broad-spectrum aerobic and anaerobic agent limited in its use by an unpredictable capacity to cause fatal aplastic anaemia in upwards of 1 in every 20,000 prescriptions. It remains important in the therapy of typhoid perforation. This apart, there are no common surgical indications now other than in neurosurgery—in particular for cerebral abscess and subdural empyema—and possibly some infections complicating vascular grafting.

Erythromycin

This is an effective drug for gram positive coccal disease and it also has significant anti-anaerobic activity. It is used for staphylococcal and streptococcal disease in patients with penicillin allergy. Usually given q.i.d. orally as 1.0–2.0 g/day, although parenteral preparations are available. The ester, erythromycin estolate, can cause a painful cholestatic hypersensitivity jaundice and should not be used.

Lincomycin and clindamycin

These drugs were initially introduced for staphylococcal disease, and a particular capacity to penetrate bone claimed, which suggested a special usefulness in osteomyelitis. Though certainly effective, it was never established that they were an improvement on older more conventional regimens. Recognition of their broad spectrum anti-anaerobic activity resulted in increasing use in the early 1970's until the potentially fatal large bowel disease (pseudomembranous colitis) became linked with their use. Although this disease, caused mostly by toxin producing *Cl. difficile*, has now been seen with *all* antibacterial drugs, and although there are very clear geographical variations in its incidence, this family of drugs has rightly retained limited use in many parts of the world because of this association.

Tetracyclines

These are broad spectrum antibiotics with aerobic and anaerobic activity, formerly used in surgery for abdominal sepsis. Resistance in both aerobic and anaerobic gram negative bacilli has diminished their use in this situation. They remain useful drugs for several important and common community infections, e.g. acute purulent exacerbations of chronic respiratory disease, acute sinusitis and sexually transmitted chlamydial infections. Doxycycline is a widely used tetracycline, 100 mg given once a day only and it lacks the major deleterious effects of earlier tetracyclines on already compromised renal function. Local use of tetracycline for abdominal lavage (1 g/L of wash solution) is currently popular and exerts its effects by a high *bactericidal* concentration. Tetracyclines are potentially nephrotoxic.

Nitrofurantoin

This drug is recommended only for bladder infections: it has no antibacterial effect other than when excreted and concentrated in urine. It is cheap and, though nausea is often a problem, low doses of 50 mg q.i.d. are as effective as the earlier more nauseating larger doses advised. The common causes of urinary tract infection remain sensitive to it.

Nystatin

This is a useful anti-candida drug. Resistance does not develop to it. It is not absorbed from the gastrointestinal tract and is most useful given for oral candidiasis as a suspension 2 hourly, initially held in the mouth and thereafter 4–6 hourly when the disease is controlled. Candida infection of the mouth is a not uncommon consequence of polyantibiotic therapy. It can lead to systemic candidiasis.

Prophylaxis

Introduction

The development of wound infection is determined at the time of operation or shortly thereafter by the implantation of organisms into the tissues. The presence of high tissue antibacterial concentrations at the time prevents multiplication and helps elimination of organisms before they reach numbers that make infection, as distinct from contamination, inevitable. The principles of prophylaxis have been established in animal models, though there is much controversy about the precise recommendations. The experimental work has shown the efficacy of:

1. Rapidly bactericidal combinations in single preoperative doses (e.g. penicillins plus aminoglycosides) OR
2. Less rapidly bactericidal drugs for a longer period beginning with a large preoperative dose.

In practice an endeavour should be made to use agents which are cheap, not used therapeutically, of low toxicity, and have low percentage resistance.

The following rules govern prophylactic therapy:

1. Use it where the risks of potential infective complications seem likely to outweigh the possible risks, costs and usage difficulties of the prophylactic drug or drugs.
2. Use drugs selected rationally with an awareness of the likely infecting organisms.
3. Begin their administration *immediately* preoperatively and do not continue for more than 24–48 hours at the most. There are some studies which show the efficacy even of *single* preoperative doses.

Endocarditis prevention

This is a special and very important area of prophylaxis. Patients with valve or other anatomical cardiac defects or prosthetic heart valves or cerebrospinal prostheses are at risk of endocarditis or infection of their shunts from bacteraemia. Dental manipulations may cause bacteraemia with streptococcus viridans and genitourinary, large bowel and gynaecological procedures may cause enterococcal (Group D streptococci, *S. faecalis*) bacteraemia. Prevention is aimed *only* at these *particular* organisms in each of these clinical settings.

Suggestions which incorporate those principles, and should provide optimal (and maximal rather than minimal) protection, are as follows:

Dental manipulations

1. Benzylpenicillin 1.2 g + gentamicin 100 mg half an hour before procedure.
2. Amoxycillin 3 g oral 1–1½ hours before procedure on an empty stomach and 6 hourly for 24 hours.
3. Erythromycin 2.0 g oral 1½–2 hours before procedure on an empty stomach and 500 mg 6 hourly for 24–48 hours.

Genitourinary, female genital tract procedures

1. Ampicillin 500 mg + gentamicin 80 mg IM/IV half an hour before procedure. Consider continuing 8 hourly for further 2 doses.
2. Vancomycin 1.0 g IV run in over the 30–45 minutes immediately before procedure + streptomycin 1.0 g IM half an hour before procedure. Consider repeating both drugs in 12 hours.

Gut—see specific recommendations on p. 162.

Prophylaxis of gas gangrene

It is negligent not to give benzylpenicillin 1.2 g 4 times daily IM to patients who are at risk of gas gangrene.

1. Large wounds involving muscle at whatever site.
2. Amputations of the lower limb in diabetics.

It is safe to assume in all circumstances that we are smeared below the pubis with a thin layer of liquid faeces.

Tuberculostatic Drugs

Specialised advice should always be sought.

Initial phase treatment—duration up to 8 weeks.:

Usual drugs	Isoniazid 300 mg daily (3 mg/kg)
	Rifampacin 450–600 mg (10 mg/kg) daily before breakfast.
and either	Ethambutol 15 mg/kg daily
or	Streptomycin 1 g daily

Continuation treatment—duration up to 1 year:

Isoniazid as above
Rifampacin, ethambutol or streptomycin as above or twice weekly.

All these agents have complex and potentially dangerous side-effects. Check the Formulary and manufacturer's literature and always seek advice.

7. CYTOTOXIC AND IMMUNOSUPPRESSIVE DRUGS

Systemic Cytotoxic Therapy

Despite the relative insensitivity of most solid tumours to chemotherapy, this method of treatment is being used with increasing frequency by surgeons, physicians, radiotherapists and medical oncologists. It is not the role of the house surgeon to determine when they should be used or in what dosage. However, he may be called upon to administer them according to a protocol and he must be aware of their side-effects (see Table 6) and the precautions that should be taken to detect these at an early stage.

Body weight and height

These should be measured before each course of therapy because dosage is based on body weight or on surface area, calculated from the ideal body weight and height.

68

Table 6 Side-effects of anti-cancer agents

Drug	Haematological	Gastrointestinal	Dermatological	Other
Actinomycin D	Thrombocytopenia, Leucopenia, anaemia.	Anorexia, nausea, vomiting, diarrhoea, proctitis, glossitis, stomatitis.	Alopecia, erythema with desquamation. Acneiform eruption. Hyperpigmentation.	Potentiates radiotherapy.
Adriamycin	Leucopenia, thrombocytopenia, anaemia.	Anorexia, nausea, vomiting, stomatitis, oesophagitis.	Alopecia. Hyperpigmentation.	Cardiotoxic. Fever.
Bleomycin		Stomatitis.	Dermatitis.	Pulmonary fibrosis. Fever.
Cis-Platinum		Anorexia, nausea, vomiting. Paralytic ileus.		Highly nephrotoxic. Also audiotoxic, vestibulotoxic, peripheral neuropathy.
Cyclophosphamide	Leucopenia, anaemia, thrombocytopenia.	Anorexia, nausea, vomiting.	Alopecia, hyperpigmentation, ridging of nails.	Haemorrhagic cystitis.
Cytosine Arabinoside	Leucopenia, anaemia, thrombocytopenia.	Anorexia, nausea, vomiting. Hepatic dysfunction.		
DTIC	Leucopenia, thrombocytopenia.	Anorexia, nausea, vomiting. Diarrhoea.	Alopecia, facial flushing.	

Drug	Haematological	Gastrointestinal	Dermatological	Other
5-Fluoro-uracil	Leucopenia, thrombocytopenia.	Anorexia, nausea, vomiting. Diarrhoea, stomatitis.	Alopecia.	
Methotrexate	Leucopenia, thrombocytopenia.	Stomatitis, diarrhoea. Hepatic dysfunction.	Alopecia, dermatitis.	Osteoporosis.
Mitomycin C	Leucopenia, thrombocytopenia.	Hepatic dysfunction.		Renal dysfunction.
Mithramycin	Leucopenia, thrombocytopenia, coagulopathy.	Nausea, vomiting. Hepatic dysfunction.		
Nitrosourea	Prolonged leucopenia, thrombocytopenia.	Anorexia, nausea, vomiting.		
Phenylalanine mustard	Prolonged leucopenia, thrombocytopenia.	Anorexia, nausea, vomiting.		
Streptozotocin		Anorexia, nausea, vomiting.		Nephrotoxic.
Thiotepa	Leucopenia, thrombocytopenia.			
Vinblastine	Leucopenia, thrombocytopenia, anaemia.	Anorexia, nausea, vomiting. Stomatitis, constipation or diarrhoea.		

Drug	Haematological	Gastrointestinal	Dermatological	Other
Vincristine		Constipation, abdominal pain.	Alopecia.	Loss of deep tendon reflexes, mild paraesthesias up to severe peripheral neuropathy. Hoarseness, ptosis, double vision.

Intravenous administration

Most agents are powerful tissue irritants. Therefore they should be given slowly in dilute solution and into as large a vein as possible. It is essential that there is no leakage into the tissue because necrosis may result. In order to be certain that the needle is inside the vein, run in normal saline/dextrose before putting the drug into the IV set. If extravasation occurs, stop the drip and aspirate back with the syringe. Inject hydrocortisone through the same needle before withdrawal. If need arises, subcutaneous hydrocortisone can also be injected. The extravasated area should be dressed well to prevent secondary infection. Some units use indwelling subclavian catheters for chemotherapy and this is recommended.

Bone marrow depression

This is the most constant side-effect. If blood counts are low the dose modification varies according to the agents being used and the protocol being followed, but the absolute granulocyte count and absolute platelet count are the most important for chemotherapy.

Control of Malignant Pleural Effusion

If there is a moderate pleural effusion which is hampering respiration it should be aspirated. A more major effusion should be drained by an intercostal tube. Several agents are used for recurrent pleural effusions. All act as chemical irritants. Some of the agents for this purpose are:

1. Mepacrine.
2. Tetracycline.
3. Nitrogen Mustard (mechlorethamine).

Mepacrine is the most commonly used drug. Before instilling it into the pleural cavity all the fluid should be drained and a tube left in situ. Three hundred mg of freshly prepared mepacrine is put into the pleural cavity through the chest drain. The tube is clamped for 4 hours and the position of the patient changed frequently. Remove the drug after 4 hours. The local instillation can be repeated for the next 2 days. Side-effects of all these agents include local pain, fever and loculated pleural effusion.

Control of Malignant Ascites

The following methods are used: Repeated drainage, diuretics, local radiotherapy, cytotoxic agents such as thiotepa, and radioactive colloids such as ^{32}P. Rarely a peritoneovenous shunt may be done.

Immunosuppression

Azathioprine

Apart from its use in organ transplantation it has been found to be of some value in Crohn's disease.
Dose: adult—100–150 mg daily.

Other imunosuppressants

Cyclosporin A is an exciting drug. Housemen may well have to come to terms with it but it is, at the time of writing, an experimental agent.

8. BLOOD TRANSFUSION

Stringent regulations for the 'consumer' are necessary to run an efficient, safe Blood Transfusion Service. For the house surgeon, special attention to blood transfusion procedures is necessary as often patients need to go to the operating room urgently, are anaesthetised, or unconscious. Under these conditions the signs of major transfusion reactions may be obscured. The following notes incorporate some guiding principles for house surgeons.

Patient Identity

There must always appear on the request form the patient's full name, age or date of birth and hospital number, his blood group (if known) and whether the person has previously been transfused, has been pregnant or has known blood group antibodies. By the same token, before each unit of blood is given to the patient, his name, hospital number and blood group must be checked with the label on the blood unit. These precautions are valueless unless it is certain that the initial blood sample taken for crossmatching has been from the correct patient and for this reason the house surgeon should either take the blood sample himself or be assured that the arrangements for blood collection are carefully checked.

Remember, most major transfusion errors result from mistakes in clerical and identification procedures.

Request for Blood

Operative procedures can be divided into 3 groups in which:

1. Blood transfusion is invariable.
2. Blood transfusion is occasional.
3. Blood transfusion is rare.

The house surgeon's aim should be on the one hand to avoid excessive demands on the Transfusion Service and on the other hand to ensure that blood is readily available when required.

These two aims can be reconciled in cases of category (1) and (2) above by

1. Sending blood for grouping and antibody screening before the patient is admitted. A good Surgical Unit will organise this in the outpatient clinic.

2. 48 hours before operation sending a further sample with the appropriate request:

(a) 'Please crossmatch X units of blood for operation on Y date.' or

(b) 'Please group, antibody screen and hold serum for 7 days.'

Crossmatching can be performed on this serum if urgently required.

The safest patient to transfuse is the patient with a negative antibody screen and who has never been transfused or had a pregnancy. Transfusion reactions in such patients, except for major ABO incompatibility, are rare.

Blood Requirements for Operation

Many hospital Blood Banks now adopt a policy of grouping, antibody screening and holding the serum for crossmatch if required and in only certain operative procedures does blood need to be actually

74

held crossmatched in the Blood Bank. *In general, blood should not be requested unless it is fairly certain that it will be used.* You should always try to inform the Blood Bank if blood that has been crossmatched is no longer required as this allows the blood to be used for another patient.

The following operations should always have blood crossmatched prior to surgery. However, check your hospital policy on this matter before ordering.

Radical or total mastectomy	2 units
Major renal surgery, nephrectomy, nephrolithotomy, partial nephrectomy	2 units
Prostatectomy, open or transurethral	2 units
Bladder surgery	2 units
Major head and neck surgery	2 units
Carotid disobliteration	2 units
Femoro-popliteal bypass or embolectomy	3 units
Aortic surgery	8 units
Oesophageal surgery	4 units
Gastric surgery	2 units
Colectomy	3 units
Abdomino-perineal resection	4 units

Thyroid surgery, needle biopsy of liver or kidney: group, antibody screen and hold serum for possible crossmatch.

The needs of other operations will be determined by your hospital policy.

In replacement of red cells prior to operation, the transfusion should be given 24–36 hours prior to surgery to enable the stored cells to recover their full oxygen carrying capacity in vivo.

Storage of Blood

All blood must be stored in properly regulated Blood Bank refrigerators. The correct temperature for the storage of blood is

4–6°C. It must never be frozen. Ward refrigerators are unsafe for the storage of blood, particularly if they have a freezing compartment into which blood may inadvertently be placed.

Once non-refrigerated units of blood have left the Blood Bank, unless they are used almost immediately, they are unsafe if the core temperature of the blood rises above 8°C. In an ambient temperature of 22°C this takes place in 30 minutes. Blood issued from the Blood Bank should be in refrigerated insulated containers and only one or two units should be issued at a time. If not used, blood must be immediately returned to the Blood Bank. If there is a delay in return of the blood to the Blood Bank the bags should be labelled 'Not for transfusion'.

Urgent Blood Transfusion

At night and at weekends the telephone operator has the name and telephone number of the member of the Blood Bank staff on duty. Much help can be given in the clinical situation if consultation is made and possible future requests are explained personally. This particularly applies in the massive transfusion situation.

The recommended procedure in a patient apparently needing urgent transfusion is:

1. Warn the Blood Bank
2. Insert IV cannula using this to take blood sample for grouping, antibody screening and crossmatching
3. Send this sample to the Blood Bank *immediately* with the request form.
4. Depending on the degree of urgency, request the Blood Bank for:
   (a) O Rh(d) negative blood—*extreme* emergency only.
   (b) Grouped but not crossmatched blood—*great* urgency, 5–10 minutes.
   (c) Grouped and saline crossmatched blood—15 minutes.
   (d) Fully crossmatched blood—1 hour.
5. In the meantime use a plasma product or substitute.

At all stages it is essential to weigh the risk of transfusion reaction against that of incomplete or improper replacement of blood loss. It is important to substitute fully crossmatched blood as soon as it becomes available.

Many hospitals now have abbreviated crossmatch procedures which allow the earlier safe issue of blood. The use of non-crossmatched blood must be kept to an absolute minimum as it is safer to have done a simple crossmatch than no crossmatch at all.

Transfusion Reactions

Transfusion reactions may be divided up into mild, moderate and severe. In mild reactions as evidenced by transient skin rashes, hives (skin urticaria) or facial oedema, treatment with antihistamines is usually sufficient. It is usual to discard the unit of blood involved and commence on a new unit and transfuse this carefully. However, all transfusion reactions should be reported to the Blood Transfusion Service.

Moderate and severe reactions

Any untoward event that occurs during transfusion (fever, rigor, back ache, shock) and which suggests incompatibility or bacterial contamination of the blood or blood products must be investigated to determine the cause.

The procedure is as follows:

1. Stop the infusion, keeping all blood units.
2. Re-check all labelling and documentation procedures.
3. Take a specimen of blood from the opposite arm to which the transfusion is given, into both plain and EDTA tubes, and send these, plus the blood units, to the Blood Bank for investigation.
4. Always consult with the Blood Bank staff and the Pathologist on call. A re-check of the documentation and a repeat check crossmatch will usually detect if a major serological incompatibility is present and the results of this finding will determine whether urgent further action is required.
5. Check the urine for the presence of free haemoglobin. It is also of use to test for the presence of free haemoglobin in the serum, a lowering of plasma haptoglobins and the presence of bilirubin.
6. Observe urinary output carefully.

In a well managed Blood Bank, major blood group serological

reactions are uncommon and most transfusion reactions appear to be due to leucocyte, platelet or serum antibodies which are often difficult to categorise. If all investigations are negative, crossmatched compatible blood can again be transfused with care, under the cover of antihistamines or a steroid if required. Pyrexic reactions which appear to have no specific cause can be treated with aspirin, but remember blood transmitted malaria.

Patients with repeated transfusion reactions, with or without demonstrable antibody present, should be managed with leucocyte poor, or washed red cells.

Severe reactions due to ABO or Rhesus incompatibility can occur and these are usually due to documentation errors. In any patient in whom severe backache, shock and haemoglobinuria are present, the use of heparin to prevent disseminated intravascular coagulation, and infusion of mannitol or intravenous frusemide to promote diuresis should be considered. Such treatment may need to be instituted urgently but in consultation with the attending Clinician and the Pathologist.

Blood Products and Plasma Substitutes

The availability and cost of these varies greatly from country to country and hospital to hospital. The pattern of usage will depend upon the overall policy of the country, availability of fractioned products and finance available.

Whole blood

Whole blood should be reserved for patients in whom there is acute blood loss and where both red cell and plasma volume replacement is essential. Whole blood should not be used for routine blood transfusion.

Packed cells

Packed cells should be used for the management of most patients who require restoration of their red cell mass and who are not actively bleeding. Many hospitals now find that over 70% of blood transfusions can be given as packed cells thus preserving plasma for further processing.

Resuspended cells

The recent introduction of red cells resuspended in an electrolyte medium reduces the haematocrit of packed cells and these are now being used in some hospitals. They reduce the problem of slow flow rate of packed cells.

Platelets

Most centres now prepare platelet concentrates which can be stored for 3 days usually at room temperature. Platelet rich plasma may also be used. Platelets must be mixed carefully during storage and kept at the correct temperature. Platelets may be used for the treatment of patients with certain forms of thrombocytopenia and particularly in haematological patients. They are useful in the perioperative period for cover for procedures such as splenectomy, porto-systemic shunts, etc. Fresh whole blood (less than 24 hours old) can sometimes be used where both a platelet and red cell defect are present.

Leucocyte poor red cells

Various methods are available for the preparation of these including centrifugation, filtration, dextran sedimentation and saline washing. For patients with repeated transfusion reactions these types of preparations are useful and need to be specially requested from the Blood Transfusion Service.

Plasma volume expanders

These can be divided into plasma substitutes and human plasma derivatives. Plasma substitutes include *dextran* (70,000), *modified gelatin* (Haemacel) and *hydroxyethyl starch* (Volex). All are commercially available and have the advantage of being emergency blood volume expanders because of their ready availability, storage characteristics, relatively low cost and freedom from the hepatitis virus. Each have their advantages and disadvantages but none is as satisfactory as derivatives of human plasma.

Plasma derivatives

Plasma protein solutions (PPS) are now used in many countries and these are obtained by fractionation of human plasma. They contain 4–5% protein mainly consisting of albumin with some globulins. The solutions are free of the hepatitis virus and have a long shelf life. As they are excellent plasma volume expanders they are used extensively in emergency situations, but are expensive in terms of original starting plasma and cost of fractionation.

Plasma

Plasma is sometimes used as a volume expander but should not be utilised when other products are available. Plasma is too valuable a product to be used in this way. However, where other substitutes are not available and hepatitis B antigen testing is satisfactory, plasma can be used.

Clotting Factors and Coagulation Defects

In surgical practice it is important to define these adequately. Patients who have a clinical or family history of a bleeding defect should always be investigated preoperatively to define the defect and it is wise to plan with a haematologist for prophylaxis against possible bleeding.

When a coagulation defect or bleeding diathesis becomes apparent in the course of an operation the advice of a haematologist may not be immediately available and empirical therapy with clotting factors has to be undertaken. It is advisable in these circumstances to use fresh frozen, or freeze-dried plasma remembering that these blood products carry a small risk of transmission of hepatitis. The dangerous situation is a massive transfusion where there may be dilution of clotting factors with subsequent bleeding and oozing.

Two defined clinical circumstances can be described:

1. In massive blood loss (ruptured aneurysm, major vascular injury, multiple injuries) or blood destruction (prolonged cardiopulmonary by-pass) when many protein clotting factors may be depleted, and there has been massive transfusion, use fresh frozen or dried plasma to restore clotting factors. Give at least 2 units initially. If whole blood is also being used ensure that it is less than 1 week old

as this reduces any problems with microaggregate formation in the transfused blood. If there is any evidence of pulmonary insufficiency a microaggregate filter may need to be used. After a transfusion of 10 units of blood there is often a depletion of platelets, thus a platelet count and clotting screen should be performed. If platelets are below $100 \times 10^3/\mu l$, platelet concentrates may be required.

2. In septicaemia, massive venous thrombosis, brain, prostatic and lung surgery and occasionally in other conditions, coagulation may be followed by excess fibrinolysis with the release of degradation products of fibrin which act as inhibitors of the intrinsic clotting cascade. Fresh frozen or freeze-dried plasma, and platelet transfusion, are usually effective as long as the primary condition is adequately treated. If clotting factors are very low, the use of cryoprecipitate to provide Factor VIII and fibrinogen may be helpful. On rare occasions an anti-fibrinolytic agent such as epsilon aminocaproic acid (EACA) or aprotinin (Trasylol) can be useful. *Consultation with a haematologist is essential for adequate management of these patients.*

9. IV FLUID THERAPY AND NUTRITION

Techniques of IV Infusion

1. Ideally an infusion should not be run into a peripheral vein for more than 24 hours—thrombophlebitis is always painful and sometimes dangerous. Change all peripheral infusions before this time. Although this is a counsel of perfection it *is* possible and in fact saves discomfort for the patient and time for the houseman in the long run. One way of accomplishing this is to use disposable 'butterfly' scalp vein sets for most peripheral infusions.

2. Technical points for peripheral infusions:
   (a) Become familiar with one piece of equipment and use it all the time.
   (b) Use the thinnest needles or cannulae compatible with the purpose.
   (c) Avoid the elbow fold—the forearm and dorsum of the hand are ideal.
   (d) Do not use the lower limb—the inevitable immobility and superficial venous thrombosis causes a risk of deep vein thrombosis and pulmonary embolism.

(e) Anaesthetise the skin before inserting a catheter. A fine intradermal weal of 1% lignocaine is ideal.

(f) Sit down to carry out the venepuncture.

(g) Use a tourniquet but do not slap the veins. A gentle tap is enough.

(h) Do not try to puncture the skin and the vein all in one movement. The skin is tough; the vein is not. Puncture the skin to one side of the vein; then take the needle over the vein and deliberately 'dip' into it.

(i) Secure the cannula yourself. Then you are to blame if it comes out.

3. Long continued infusions are now relatively commonplace, mainly to carry out intravenous feeding or 'parenteral alimentation' as it is usually called. A very large variety of cannulae are available which can be inserted in such a way as to lie in a central vein (usually the brachiocephalic or superior vena cava) so that the administered substances are rapidly diluted by the flow of blood. A long catheter can be led up to the deep veins by percutaneous puncture of the basilic or external jugular. The disadvantage of the first is that the arm is immobilised; of the second, that negotiating the junction of the external and internal jugular veins can be difficult, if not impossible. For these reasons the site of choice is now usually the subclavian below the clavicle. Whether done by percutaneous puncture or direct exposure, this is a job for an expert as the complications are almost endless. Rules to be observed are:

(a) Always take an X-ray after insertion to ensure correct placement
   (i) within the vein
   (ii) in relation to the chambers of the heart
   (iii) to detect the occasional instance when the catheter wanders over to the other side or into the internal jugular vein.

(b) Take a twice weekly blood culture.

(c) Remove the catheter if there is a spike of fever unexplained by any other cause. Culture the tip when you do.

(d) In some units there is a policy of changing the catheter routinely every 7–10 days. However, catheters which are well looked after can stay in for months. If the catheter is to be removed this means complete removal and re-insertion on the opposite side—not threading a new catheter over a guide wire inserted through the old one.

(e) Constantly exhort the nursing staff to the highest standards of sterile procedure in changing bottles. Do not let infusion sets stay unchanged if there is the slightest sign of contamination or if thick liquids such as fat emulsions or blood have been used.

(f) Change the dressing at the site of puncture every second day, cleaning the area with an alcoholic antiseptic such as chlorhexidine. Do not use antibiotic creams because these encourage superinfection.

4. If a patient is to undergo a major operation or a rapid blood transfusion, a catheter of at least 4 mm external diameter should be inserted into an arm vein. Usually this can be done by percutaneous puncture, preferably away from the elbow flexure; it is a kindness to use local anaesthetic infiltration or to wait until general anaesthesia has been induced (this usually makes the chosen vein an easier target).

5. It is rare nowadays that it is necessary to cut down on a vein. However, patients in shock with a tightly constricted circulation or those with a need for massive transfusion should have a large cannula inserted by exposing a vein in the antecubital fossa. This is preferable to multiple unsuccessful attempts to puncture a vein while the situation is deteriorating. Full aseptic precautions must be observed whenever a cut down is undertaken.

Intravenous Solutions

We favour the use of simple solutions to which other ingredients can be added, or which can be rendered hypertonic by the addition of an ampoule of a concentrate, rather than complex solutions. However, in circumstances where very large quantities of intravenous fluid are required (e.g. burns), Hartmann's solution may be preferred as the basic solution, rather than 'normal' saline. The electrolyte content and approximate energy value of various solutions are given below:

'Normal' saline	Na^+	150 mmol/1
	Cl'	150 mmol/1
5% dextrose	Calories:	180/1
Hypotonic ('⅕th normal')	Na^+	30 mmol/1
saline	Cl'	30 mmol/1
and 4% dextrose	Calories:	140/1

'Normal' sodium lactate	$\begin{cases} Na^+ & 150 \text{ mmol/l} \\ Lactate' & 150 \text{ mmol/l} \end{cases}$
'Normal' sodium bicarbonate	Na^+ 150 mmol/l HCO_3' 150 mmol/l
20% dextrose	Calories: 700/l
50% dextrose	Calories: 1800/l
20% KCl	10 ml = 2 g KCl $\backsimeq$ 25 mmol K^+
Hartmann's balanced salt solution	$\begin{cases} Na^+ & 131 \text{ mmol/l} \\ K^+ & 5 \text{ mmol/l} \\ Ca^{++} & 4 \text{ mmol/l} \\ Cl' & 111 \text{ mmol/l} \\ Lactate' & 29 \text{ mmol/l} \end{cases}$
Concentrated sodium chloride	Usually supplied as 2, 3, or 4 times 'normal'

Alimentary Secretions

As a working rule, the secretions of the alimentary tract can be considered to contain Na^+ 130 mmol/l, K^+ 10 mmol/l, i.e. so far as these cations are concerned each litre lost from the body as vomit, gastrointestinal aspirate, diarrhoea, or from an alimentary fistula may be replaced by a litre of 'normal' saline containing at least 12.5 mmol of K^+.

The situation with regard to anions is more variable: bile, pancreatic juice and small-gut secretions contain large quantities of HCO_3', while gastric juice contains large quantities of Cl'. In practice, adequate renal function may be assumed to regulate the Cl'/HCO_3' balance, and gastro-intestinal losses may be replaced litre for litre by 'normal' saline containing 12.5 mmol K^+/l.

Electrolyte and Water Balance Techniques

So-called 'fluid balance' is potentially one of the most abused techniques in hospital practice. The routine prescription of 'fluid balance chart' by the house surgeon presupposes that the keeping of such a balance is of equal importance in all patients for whom it is prescribed, and that the nursing staff are able to achieve perfection in all such patients.

It is important to set two standards of accuracy—routine and special:

Routine. Here an accurate record of the *volume and nature of the 24-hour* oral and IV fluid intake, and *24-hour volume of urine* excreted is required:

1. Prescriptions for IV water and electrolyte therapy and for nutrition (p. 98) should be arranged in the early morning (6–8 a.m.) to achieve consistency of balance studies. Always prescribe each day's IV requirement in legible writing (preferably printing) and on night rounds make sure that the nurse understands it. It eliminates confusion and saves you being woken at night.
2. When a drip fails in the middle of the night, it is only permissible to wait till morning to replace it if the patient is having *maintenance therapy*. When *replacement therapy* is in progress the drip must be attended to whatever the hour.
3. Measurement of daily *urine output* by the standard method of measuring and recording each volume passed is adequate. In an adult, provided it exceeds 1 litre daily from the second day after operation, and there are no excessive losses, the patient may be considered to be in balance.
4. Haematocrit, blood urea, serum creatinine, Na^+, K^+, and HCO_3' concentrations to be estimated every 2 days.

Special. This is applied only in complicated cases and must be watched meticulously. *Nothing less than perfection is adequate.*

1. *IV or oral requirements* are prescribed in writing for each 24-hour period. If possible, the patient should be put in a single room so that the traffic of fluid in and out can be more easily controlled. It is best if you personally label the prescribed bottles with the patient's name and number them in sequence. They can be placed by the patient's bed with instructions that none are to be removed, used or unused, until they are checked by you or Sister at the end of the period.
2. For each 24-hour period, all *urine* passed is placed without measurement in a container. At the end of the period the

24-hour volume is measured by you or Sister. An *aliquot* is then placed in a specimen bottle and the Na^+ and K^+ measured (and on occasions urea concentration and SG) by the laboratory.

3. All *gastric aspirate*, vomit or other losses are placed in a second container and the volume is also measured at the end of the period and an aliquot sent for Na^+ and K^+ estimation.

4. The patient should be *weighed daily* using either an accurate chair balance or a bed-weighing machine. This technique is more honoured in the breach than in the observance, but is extremely useful.

5. Haematocrit, blood urea, serum creatinine, Na^+ and K^+ to be estimated each day and the results charted as a graph. Arterial blood pH, pCO_2, base deficit or standard bicarbonate and serum protein (albumin) may sometimes be required.

Intravenous Fluid Regimens

It is important to distinguish the three situations in which water, electrolytes and a source of calories are administered intravenously.

Maintenance therapy implies that there are no unusual external losses, so that merely the normal daily requirements are administered. This is not a strictly accurate description of the immediate postoperative period, for there may be hidden losses, but this period will nevertheless be considered under the heading of maintenance.

Replacement of continuing losses is necessary when there is excessive loss from the gastrointestinal or urinary tracts. These losses are usually roughly measurable, so the task of replacement is a relatively easy one.

Replacement of past losses is much more difficult, for there is no way of precisely measuring how great these losses have been. A first estimate can be made of their magnitude by a combination of clinical acumen and biochemical measurement, but complete replacement is achieved by successive approximation. A sub-set of this category is the correction of *acid-base disturbances*, and this topic will be treated separately.

Maintenance therapy

The daily maintenance requirements for a resting normal adult in a temperate climate are, in the medium term, approximately:

Na^+	90 mmol
K^+	75 mmol
Calories	1500 (6300J)
Water	2500 ml

These can be provided only by the use of complex solutions or mixtures of solutions which, because of the caloric requirement, are hypertonic and so must be given into a central vein. Moreover, in the perioperative period this prescription is no longer valid (see Table 6), and for very long-term maintenance other cations such as Ca^{++} and Mg^{++} are necessary, as well as a variety of trace elements. Thus we recommend, as a compromise, that a sequence of three maintenance regimens be employed for: the first 1–2 postoperative days; the next 3–5 days; and for the longer-term, should this be necessary.

First 1–2 postoperative days. During this time there are two disturbances of water and electrolyte handling which have a bearing on maintenance requirements. On the one hand, the kidney's ability to excrete a water and sodium load is restricted because of the influence of ADH (vasopressin) and aldosterone. On the other hand, there are continuing losses into and around the operative site: damaged capillaries 'leak' a plasma ultrafiltrate into the tissues and serous cavities, and (especially after abdominal operations) there may be sequestration of extracellular fluid into the bowel lumen. Both processes depend on the duration and magnitude of the operation.

An approximate guide to fluid and electrolyte maintenance requirements in the first 1–2 postoperative days is set out in Table 7. It should be emphasised that the regimen takes no account of abnormal external losses, which must be provided for in addition (see Replacement of Continuing Losses, p. 89). It should also be emphasised that the regimens assume that there is adequate renal function. After very major operations neither the assumption nor the predictions may be accurate. Thus, it should be noted that on postoperative days 1–5 we have prescribed sodium in excess of the normal daily requirements: this is to allow for concealed losses and presupposes normal renal function.

Postoperative days 3–5. During this period it can be anticipated that the sequestered water and electrolytes will be progressively released, and so be available for redistribution in the extracellular space or for

Table 7 Peroperative maintenance regimens (70 kg adult)

Magnitude of operation	Average requirements
Minor: hernia, peripheral orthopaedic, uncomplicated appendicectomy	Oral fluids only
Medium: cholecycstectomy, vagotomy, hiatus hernia	Peroperative: 1l Hartmann's Day 1: 1l Hartmann's, 1l 5% dextrose Day 2: 1l Hartmann's, 2l 5% dextrose
Major: gastrectomy, colectomy, hip replacement	Peroperative: 1l Hartmann's Day 1: 2l Hartmann's, 1l 5% dextrose Day 2: 1l Hartmann's, 2l 5% dextrose
Maximal: oesophagectomy, abdomino-perineal resection, open-heart surgery	Peroperative: 2l Hartmann's Day 1: 2l Hartmann's, 1l 5% dextrose Day 2: 1l Hartmann's 2l 5% dextrose

excretion. At the same time the ability of the kidney to excrete a salt and water load returns towards normal, so that there is a greater safety-margin.

In the previous 2 days the patient has been provided with adequate Na^+ and water (and indeed is likely to be in positive balance), but with few calories. K^+ intake has been low, but there will have been release of K^+ from cells. Thus up to a deadline of the end of the 5th postoperative day we advise the daily maintenance intravenous intake be:

1l Hartmann's solution
2l 5% dextrose

The 5 day deadline must be a strict one: either the patient is then able to manage a normal oral intake, or intravenous feeding by way of a central venous catheter is instituted.

Postoperative day 6 onwards. If continued intravenous maintenance is required, it should be by central venous catheter. The patient is by now in negative K^+, nitrogen and energy balance, and this must not be allowed to continue. Details of intravenous nutrition are given on pp. 96–101.

It is sufficient to emphasise here that over the first few days of intravenous nutrition in such a postoperative patient the recipe should allow for K^+ depletion by providing 50–75 mmol of K^+ daily.

Replacement therapy

In addition to the maintenance requirements described above, external losses through drains, fistulae, gastric aspirate or vomitus must be replaced. These are susceptible to accurate volume-measurement, so that in the short term they can be replaced by an equal volume of a solution containing approximately Na^+ 150 mmol/l, K^+ 10 mmol/l. Hartmann's solution has the virtue of being commercially available, but contains only 5 mmol K^+/l. We therefore still prefer to use a composite solution for replacement: 1l of 'normal saline' (Na^+ 150 mmol/l) plus 5 ml of 20% KCl/l (K^+ 12.5 mmol/l).

There are two other circumstances in which replacement therapy may be necessary. The postoperative maintenance regimen described above caters only for normal postoperative conditions: when abdominal distension from ileus or obstruction occurs additional, concealed losses into the bowel lumen must be counted. Further, it has so far been assumed that renal function is normal: high output (polyuric) renal failure results in substantial losses of water and electrolytes which must be replaced on a basis of the urine volume in excess of 1500 ml daily, and the measured daily excretion of Na^+ and K^+.

Replacement of past losses; water and electrolyte lack

Three classical situations are commonly encountered:

Water lack

Causes: Reduced intake from any cause; continued loss by urine (as in diabetes insipidu) and insensible routes.

Effects: The body dries out, and the patient has thirst, restlessness, hyperthermia, dry mucous membranes, and oliguria. There is an absence of circulatory disturbance because loss is evenly distributed through the whole body water.

Diagnosis. History of low intake or increased insensible loss; oliguria with high specific gravity; high plasma Na^+ and osmolality.

Correction. Water by mouth or intragastric tube; IV 5% dextrose.

Control. Monitor thirst, mucous membranes, urine volume, plasma Na^+ and osmolality. In the early postoperative period antidiuresis may keep urine volume low despite adequate replacement, but adequate perioperative fluid intake should prevent this occurring.

Sodium and water lack

Causes. Diversion of normal body secretions from GI tract, kidney or sweat glands.

Effects. The loss can be regarded as approximately isotonic with the extracellular space, so the latter shrinks without much tendency for water to be transferred from the intracellular compartment. Thus the patient develops low plasma volume and haemoconcentration, with the corresponding signs of hypovolaemia: hypotension, low CVP, oliguria. If loss has been slow there may have been water replacement and low plasma Na^+. This is *not* characteristic of acute disturbances.

Diagnosis. History of loss by vomiting, diarrhoea, fistula or polyuria; signs of hypovolaemia with empty veins, hypotension, low CVP and oliguria; usually no change in plasma electrolytes (but blood urea concentration is raised).

Correction. Replacement with normal saline or Hartmann's solution. It should be noted, however, that profound prolonged, polyuria may result in deficiency of electrolytes other than Na^+, e.g. K^+, Mg^{++}, phosphate.

Control. Monitor blood pressure, pulse rate, CVP, urine output.

Potassium lack

Causes. Overt losses from the same causes as for sodium lack; in addition starvation, sodium restriction, and diuretics may cause losses of up to 500 mmol K^+ in 10 days.

Effects. Patient inattentive, weak, depressed and sleepy; adynamic ileus; ECG changes. These may all be exaggerated by accompanying alkalosis (e.g. pyloric stenosis, diuretic therapy). Up to 500 mmol K^+ can be lost without change in plasma K^+.

Diagnosis. From causes and effects. Plasma K^+ is a poor guide, though low K^+ usually indicates severe depletion.

Treatment. Usually best to establish urine output of 30–50 ml/h by correcting Na^+ and water depletion before giving K^+. Add no more than 25 mmol K^+ to each litre of fluid except in unusual circumstances. Do not give more than 100 mmol/24 h unless, first, a good urine volume is established and, second, adequate 8 hour control of serum levels can be obtained. Sudden large infusions of K^+ may be extremely dangerous.

Control. Monitor by observation of patient, ECG, and plasma K^+. Frequency of observations depend on rate of administration of K^+. However, it should be noted that monitoring serves mainly to detect hyperkalaemia: total body K^+ depletion may be present despite a normal level of serum K^+.

Acid-Base Disturbances

Of all the aspects of pre- and post-operative management this is one of the most difficult to understand because of the mystique that still surrounds the methods of measurement and the graphical display of results. The houseman will have to learn the particular way in which results are expressed in his own hospital, but the following general guide may be useful in that all other systems can be derived from it.

The body can be looked upon as analogous to a test-tube containing a dilute solution of electrolytes in water. The alveolus is the space above the solution. Increasing or decreasing the partial pressure of CO_2 in the alveolar space increases or decreases the hydrogen ion concentration (strictly speaking 'activity', but the distinction is not important in clinical practice) in the solution because of the equilibrium:

$$CO_2 + H_2O \rightleftharpoons H_2CO_3 \rightleftharpoons H^+ + HCO_3'$$

The relationship is a linear one so that a plot of pCO_2 against hydrogen ion concentration is a straight line. In man it appears that there are two straight lines—one for pCO_2 less than normal (40 mm Hg), and one for pCO_2 greater than normal. The 95% confidence limits for normality over a wide range of pCO_2 are shown in the accompanying figure, p. 94 (a conversion table of pH into H^+ appears at the top). It follows that if pCO_2 and pH are measured in arterial blood and are found to intersect within these lines the patient is either normal (pH = 7.36; pCO_2 = 40), has a respiratory alkalosis (low pCO_2, low H^+), or a respiratory acidosis (high pCO_2, correspondingly high H^+).

If more hydrogen ions are added to the test-tube the hydrogen ion concentration for a given pCO_2 will be greater than expected from the graph. The plotted point will therefore lie to the right of the confidence limits (metabolic acidosis). If hydrogen ions are lost from the system, the plot will move to the left (metabolic alkalosis). The diagnosis for the individual patient can thus be made with precision.

The bicarbonate scale to the right of the figure is constructed so that for a given pCO_2 and H^+ the actual bicarbonate can be read off the scale. This is helpful because it is easy to see that if a patient has, say, a metabolic acidosis it is possible to determine what the actual bicarbonate concentration is and *what it should be for the same pCO_2*. The difference then gives a way of approximating the first dose of bicarbonate for correction, because the concentration deficit multiplied by the volume of the extra-cellular water (ECF) is the total compositional deficit. This dose is usually found to be less than that finally required, even if (as is not often the case in surgical patients) more hydrogen ions are not being continually added to the system. This is because using the ECF volume underestimates the volume of distribution of bicarbonate. However, in handling a situation of this kind it is better to proceed by serial approximation.

The purist may object that this account neglects the blood as a buffer system. This is so, but for practical management of the whole patient the above is a better approach as the volume of ECF greatly exceeds that of the blood and equilibrium of CO_2 thus takes place predominantly in a watery medium.

Summary of procedure

1. Draw an arterial sample and measure pCO_2 and pH.
2. Convert pH to H^+ using table of equivalent values.
3. Plot pCO_2 and H^+.
4. If within confidence limits, the patient has not got a significant metabolic component to his problem.
5. Given there is not a metabolic component it only remains to take appropriate steps to correct a high or low pCO_2 by altering alveolar ventilation.
6. If metabolic acidosis exists: use chart to determine
   (a) actual bicarbonate
   (b) bicarbonate that would exist were there a normal H^+ for the pCO_2.
7. (b—a) multiplied by 15 is a first approximation for the dose of bicarbonate required to correct the acidosis in a 70 kg adult. For larger or smaller patients use (b—a) multiplied by $0.2 \times$ body weight in kg, or figures in Appendix IV.
8. Correction of metabolic alkalosis can be accomplished in the same way using ammonium chloride solutions. However, the circumstances in which alkalosis arises in surgical patients in such a way as to require this to be done are rare and complicated (e.g. liver failure), and the acid-base imbalance is best managed by correction of the underlying problem.

The alternative way of expressing acid base problems is by taking the patient's blood and bringing it into equilibrium with gas mixtures of known composition. The results so obtained which are recorded in Appendix III represent the behaviour of blood from the patient rather than of his whole body. However, the differences are not so great as to make a practical difference in therapy. The bicarbonate deficits (acidosis) or excesses (alkalosis) are expressed as negative and positive 'base excesses' under this system and are approximately the same as those calculated from Figure 1 on p. 94.

pH	0	1	2	3	4	5	6	7	8	9
7.0	99	97	95	93	91	89	87	85	83	81
7.1	79	78	76	74	72	71	69	68	66	65
7.2	63	62	60	59	58	56	55	54	53	51
7.3	50	49	48	47	46	45	44	43	42	41
7.4	40	39	38	37	36	35	35	34	33	32
7.5	31	30	30	30	29	28	28	27	26	26
7.6	25	25	24	23	23	22	22	21	21	20
7.7	20	20	19	19	18	18	17	17	17	16
7.8	16	15	15	15	14	14	14	13	13	13
7.9	13	12	12	12	11	11	11	11	10	10

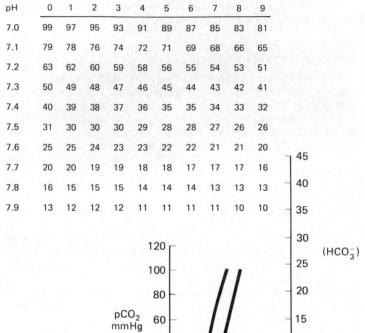

Figure 1

'Blood gases'. When a sample is drawn from an artery for pH and pCO_2 determinations it is usual to obtain the pO_2 value at the same time. This is partly because the association between acid-base disturbance and ventilation is common and partly because the apparatus is designed to give the three answers as a routine. The combined interpretation of pH, pCO_2 and pO_2 is considered on p. 104.

Oliguria and Anuria

Oliguria is arbitrarily defined as a urine output of less than 400 ml daily, and anuria a volume of less than 200 ml daily. These may be due to pre-renal factors, e.g. hypovolaemia; intrinsic renal disease, e.g. acute tubular necrosis; or obstruction. Absolute anuria (*no* urine) is rare, and usually is caused by obstruction. It should be noted that acute renal failure, or partial obstruction, may be associated with a normal or increased urine output (polyuric renal failure).

When oliguria or anuria occurs, the following procedure is instituted.

1. Assess *hydration* and *blood volume* status. Consider urinary tract obstruction.

2. Personally measure *SG* of the first urine available, and arrange or undertake *microscopic* examination. SG around 1010 and the presence of red cells, white cells or casts confirms renal damage. SG greater than 1020, in the absence of sugar or protein, suggests that pre-renal factors are responsible.

3. Institute a specially *accurate fluid balance*, record.

4. Estimate baseline *haemotocrit, blood urea, serum creatinine* and *proteins*, serum *Na⁺ and K⁺*. Also estimate *urine urea and creatinine*, osmolality and electrolytes. Pre-renal failure is suggested by a low urine Na^+ (less than 20 mmol/l), and a high urine: serum ratio of urea (over 20:1) or creatinine (over 40:1) concentrations. High urine Na^+, or low urine: serum ratios of urea and creatinine suggest intrinsic renal failure.

5. An attempt can be made to provoke an osmotic or pharmacological diuresis, to distinguish physiological from pathological oliguria. Before this is done, any blood volume or ECF deficit must be corrected. *Either* 80 mg of frusemide *or* 50 ml of 20% mannitol is given IV over 15 minutes. If 80 mg of frusemide has no effect, a larger dose, up to 500 mg IV, may be given. In physiological oliguria

the resultant urine flow, collected by catheter, should exceed 40 ml/hour.

During or following low blood pressure states frusemide or mannitol may also be given, in an attempt to avert persistent oliguria.

Management of established renal oliguria or anuria

General surgical patients can rarely be managed by oral intake techniques. Therefore:

1. The *renal physician* is consulted at the outset.
2. Basic *fluid intake is restricted* to that which covers insensible losses i.e. 600 ml/24 hours.
3. Additional *water and electrolyte losses* are replaced (including urine).
4. *Daily* haematocrit, blood urea, serum creatinine, Na^+, K^+, Cl' and base deficit or standard bicarbonate are measured.
5. The patient should be *weighed* accurately each day, and should lose 0.2–0.3 kg daily.

Before the blood urea rises above 30 mmol/l, the patient's general condition deteriorates, or the water and electrolyte state becomes seriously unbalanced, dialysis is indicated. In practice, surgical patients are in such a catabolic state that dialysis is usually established early.

Nutrition

Many surgical patients suffer from protein energy malnutrition during the course of their illness. This is thought to be significant when more than 15% of body weight has been lost, i.e. 10 kg or more below well weight in the average surgical patient. Although this degree of weight loss indicates that rehabilitation will be prolonged it is not otherwise dangerous unless associated with body protein depletion. A diagnosis of protein depletion can be made when there is evidence of wasted skeletal muscle bellies and a low level of plasma albumin. Plasma albumin, when less than 30 g/l is associated with dysfunction of many organ systems, particularly the immune system.

Nutritional assessment

When making a diagnosis of significant protein energy malnutrition it is important to remember that it is not the amount of fat and protein that has been lost that matters but how much of these stores remain.

Static nutritional assessment. All patients being admitted for major surgery should have their nutritional state assessed. The aim is to find out how much weight has been lost and what remains of the stores of body fat and protein. Thus a careful history of food intake over the month prior to admission is taken. If only half the normal intake of food has been taken over this time then more than 5 kg of body weight will have been lost. Evidence for increased energy output such as fever, vomiting or diarrhoea should also be sought. After the patient's well weight has been ascertained he is weighed and the total weight loss is calculated. Fat stores are assessed by palpation of the fat folds overlying the biceps and triceps muscles. Protein stores are assessed by palpating the temporalis, spinati, interossei, biceps and triceps muscles as well as estimating the level of plasma albumin.

Dynamic nutritional assessment. This is done by weekly measurements of body weight and plasma albumin. When the total weight loss exceeds 10 kg (and physical examination confirms that serious erosion of body fat and muscle has occurred) and especially if the plasma albumin level is less than 30 g/l then nutritional treatment is indicated.

Treatment of protein energy malnutrition

Enteral feeding. Although a skilled dietician can sometimes improve protein and energy intake in patients in whom the gastrointestinal tract is functioning, the therapeutic impact is frequently disappointing. In most patients where nutritional support is indicated and the gastrointestinal tract is functioning, the administration of a defined formula liquid diet through a fine bore nasogastric tube (Keofeed or Clinifeed tube) proves to be very satisfactory. The diet is infused continuously day and night and the most satisfactory results are obtained when a volumetric infusion pump is used. It is advisable to introduce the feeding regimen gradually to allow the patient to develop a tolerance to it and to minimise side effects. As a rough guide, 2 l of half strength feed can be given in the first 24 hours and the volume and concentration are gradually increased over the following 3 or 4 days until 3 l of the full strength feed is given in 24 hours. It is important to monitor patients daily on enteral feeding; this is done by recording accurate input and output, daily weight and blood sugar and urea creatinine and electrolytes as indicated.

Parenteral feeding. Patients requiring nutritional therapy in whom the gastrointestinal tract is *fistulated*, *blocked*, *too short*, *inflamed* or *cannot cope*, will need intravenous nutrition.

1. The Nutrient Solution. The simplest regimen is a nutrient solution made up in the pharmacy and packaged in a 3 litre plastic bag. The solution contains 1 kcal/ml and has a calorie to nitrogen ratio of around 150:1. Dextrose provides the energy source and a synthetic amino acid solution the nitrogen source. (See also Table 8.)

Table 8 Composition of 1 litre of standard solution (500 ml 8.5% crystalline amino acid plus 500 ml 50% dextrose)

Volume	1000 ml
Calories	1000 kcal
Dextrose	250 g
Amino acids	42.5 g
Nitrogen	6.25 g

Additions to each unit of base solution (average adult)

Sodium (chloride and/or acetate, lactate, bicarbonate)	40–50 mmol
Potassium (acetate, lactate, chloride, acid phosphate)	30–40 mmol
Magnesium (sulphate)	2–4 mmol
Phosphate (potassium acid salt)	6–9 mmol

Additions to only one unit daily:

Vitamin A	5000–10 000 U.S.P.	units
Vitamin D	500–1000 U.S.P.	units
Vitamin E	2.5–5.0 i.u.	

Vitamin C	250–500	mg
Thiamine	25–50	mg
Riboflavin	5–10	mg
Pyridoxine	7.5–15	mg
Niacin	50–100	mg
Pantothenic acid	12.5–25	mg
Calcium (gluconate)	2.4 – 4.8	mmol

Optional additions to daily nutrient regimen:

Vitamin K	5–10	mg	
Vitamin B_{12}	10–30	μg	
Folic acid	0.5–1.0	mg	Alternatively may be
Iron	2.0–3.0	mg	given in appropriate
Zinc	1.0–2.0	mg	weekly dosages.

Modified formulations may be required for patients with profound protein energy malnutrition (keep sodium intake very low), cardiac, renal and hepatic disease; diabetes mellitus (add insulin to nutrient solution) and other underlying diseases.

Changes in sodium, potassium, magnesium and the addition of insulin are made from day-to-day if necessary according to the information derived from the daily monitoring. These changes are ordered through the pharmacy.

2. Additives. At the beginning of the course of nutrition the patient should receive:

Vitamin B_{12} 1000 μg IM
Folic acid 15 mg IM
Vitamin K, 20 mg IM
1 bottle of 10% soybean fat emulsion via a peripheral vein

The patient may also require administration of:

A soybean fat emulsion weekly to prevent essential fatty acid deficiency
Iron for iron deficiency
Insulin for persistent hyperglycaemia
Vitamin K, folic acid and vitamin B_{12} if not supplied in the nutrient solution.

3. Requirements. Most general surgical patients will gain body protein and fat with a regimen of 50 kcal per kg body weight per day at a calorie to nitrogen ratio of 150:1.

4. Delivery. Delivery of the nutrient solution is made directly via a single line through a subclavian catheter into the superior vena cava. No Y junction or other entry is permitted to this line which is inviolate. If it is used to measure central venous pressure or for any other purpose it can no longer be used for intravenous nutrition. For this reason all additional fluids are given by separate IV infusions. The catheter is inserted and maintained according to the strict instructions set out on p. 82. Whenever there is an unexplained fever the catheter is withdrawn and not replaced for at least 12 hours.

It is usual to administer about half the calculated requirements for the first 1 or 2 days of intravenous nutrition until patient tolerance to the solution is obtained. Many complications can be avoided by controlling or correcting cardiovascular instability and metabolic derangements before commencing hyperalimentation.

Complications
    Sepsis (due to contamination of solution, tubing or catheter)
    Catheter misplacement
    Hyperglycaemia
    Volume, concentration and compositional imbalances
    Metabolic: hyperchloraemic acidosis
                 hypophosphataemia
                 trace element deficiency

Rules for monitoring
1. Observe all rules for central venous catheters—when in doubt remove catheter and replace the next day.

2. Measure body weight daily. If daily increase is greater than 0.3 kg then water is accumulating. If there is a persistent fall in body weight the patient is in negative nitrogen balance.

3. Measure plasma sodium, potassium, chloride, phosphorous, and glucose daily until patient is stable.

4. Measure liver function tests, Ca^{++}, Mg^{++}, albumin, and haemoglobin twice weekly.

5. Measure urine output daily.

6. Measure urine glucose concentration every 6 hours.

7. Carry out a weekly therapy check to avoid the all too easy mistake of carrying on a drug treatment instruction which has become unnecessary.

10 ADRENAL CORTICOIDS IN RELATION TO SURGERY

There are a limited number of situations where these are used in general surgery:

1. To provide adrenal corticoid **replacement** or **supplement** in
(a) Bilateral total adrenalectomy.
(b) In a patient undergoing operation or becoming ill who is receiving or has recently received adrenal steroid, steroid substitutes or ACTH.

N.B. It has become of great importance to question closely any patients who could have had corticoids, and who present for surgery, as to their past or present treatment, e.g. in rheumatoid arthritis, ulcerative colitis, asthma and many less probable diseases (see p. 192).

2. As a recognised *therapeutic* measure in such conditions as ulcerative colitis.

3. Rarely, as a *blind therapeutic* measure in low blood pressure states.

Replacement and Supplement

It is vital that **full absorption** be assured, so the drug must be given IV or IM if oral absorption is doubtful. Oral and IV steroids work immediately. IM route provides a reservoir and acts slowly. Use IV or IM hydrocortisone or prednisolone, whose preparations are water-soluble and even in large doses cause little salt retention.

5 mg prednisolone =   25 mg cortisol (hydrocortisone)
    or prednisone   or cortisone

Dosage schedule (as hydrocortisone):

Evening before operation	100 mg IM
Day of operation	100 mg IM b.d.
plus, during operation	100–300 mg IV
First postoperative day	100 mg IM b.d.
Then 3 days	50 mg b.d.
3 days	25 mg b.d.

Then

Replacement   **Supplement**

Start permanent maintenance   3 days 12.5 mg b.d. then stop
dose of cortisone, 12.5 to 25 mg
b.d.

plus fludrocortisone 0.1 mg
daily.

N.B. (a) If in either situation a postoperative complication such as
infection should occur, it is important to maintain the dose
of *at least* 100 mg daily till recovery.
(b) BP readings are probably the best early check on inadequate corticoid dosage. They should be made half-hourly for
the first 48 hours and thereafter 4 to 6 hourly. If hypotension persists, estimate electrolytes in blood and correct any
deficiency, especially low sodium.

Therapeutic

Therapy may be *local* or *systemic*.

Local

Hydrocortisone hemisuccinate
100 mg in 100 ml of saline.
or Prednisolone
20 mg in 100 ml of saline or as disposable enema.
Given once or twice daily as a retention enema, the foot of the
bed being elevated for 1 hour after administration.

Systemic

Prednisone or prednisolone, oral, IV or IM up to 40 mg daily.

Blind Therapeutic

Occasionally, in low blood pressure states not improved by restoration of normal blood volume and pressor agents, cortisol 250–500 mg IV may correct the situation. This should never be done without full consultation. (See p. 108.)

11 POSTOPERATIVE COMPLICATIONS

Postoperative complications will not be considered exhaustively. Only important general complications not covered elsewhere under specific headings will be mentioned.

Respiratory Complications

The likelihood of respiratory complications is much increased if the patient comes to operation with purulent sputum because of chronic bronchitis, or has not been instructed in breathing and coughing by a competent physiotherapist (see preoperative check list p. 15). Postoperative chest complications usually follow the sequence of under-ventilation—collapse—infection. It is important to recognise the stage of collapse, so often responsible for fever in the first 24 hours after operation, and to institute active *breathing and coughing exercises*. Isoprenaline aerosol may help. If significant collapse continues, *bronchosopy* may be necessary. Antibiotics are withheld unless there is definite clinical and radiological evidence of *pneumonia*, when sputum is sent for culture, and pending the result, penicillin or ampicillin are used.

It is important to remember the value of *positive pressure ventilation*, which is only successful when undertaken early rather than late. In the first instance, this should be given by way of a cuffed *endotracheal tube*. *Tracheostomy* is necessary only after several days' intubation.

The possibility of apparent *bronchopneumonia* being actually due to *embolisation* must always be considered.

In the older patient, or one from a developing country, remember *pulmonary tuberculosis*—if the chest film is suspicious, *isolate* the patient till the sputum is proven negative. These patients present a danger to the nursing and medical staff.

When collapse-consolidation occurs in the surgical patient and also on occasion when lung is put out of action in the context of trauma the changes seen in the blood gases are not those of 'medical' respiratory failure which are characteristically a low pO_2 and a high pCO_2 as a result of hypoventilation. In the surgical patient the collapsed areas produce a right to left shunt with arterial hypoxia. Further, there is rapid shallow respiration because of pain. Both these factors produce a *low* pCO_2 so that the combination usually seen in the surgical patient is a low pCO_2 and a low pO_2. Arterial pO_2 values must always be interpreted in relation to the level of inspired oxygen. A useful guide is to divide the arterial pO_2 by the fractional content of oxygen in the inspired gas. The result should be a figure exceeding 300 unless there is severe shunting.

The level of pO_2 must be interpreted against the pO_2/saturation diagram (see Figure 2). Some degree of hypoxaemia is common after major surgery and anaesthesia because of changes in distribution of inspired air in the lungs and the phenomenon of closing of small airways. If the patient's arterial oxygen tension is initially normal, the shape of the dissociation curve is such that a reduction of pO_2 to 60 mmHg is not associated with desaturation. However, if he comes to operation with borderline pO_2 then any further reduction leads to precipitate desaturation which can be of serious significance in terms of oxygen transport. It is not possible to remember this relationship and consequently it is bad medicine to 'eyeball' pO_2 figures. Always check these against the diagram and if the patient is on the steep part of the curve ask the questions:

Does a danger exist of further sputum retention, collapse or change in respiratory function from some other cause (muscle fatigue, further surgery) which could precipitate desaturation? If so what measures can I take to minimise the risk?

There is usually little danger in the use of oxygen therapy in the surgical patient because of the lack of a tendency for CO_2 retention. If there is any question of hypoxaemia in the immediate postoperative period oxygen should be administered through a venturi mask

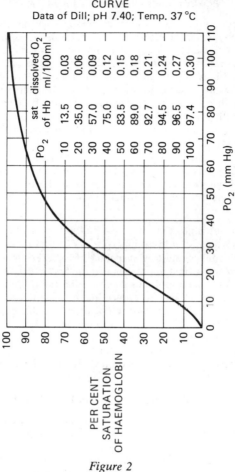

OXYGEN HAEMOGLOBIN DISSOCIATION
CURVE
Data of Dill; pH 7.40; Temp. 37 °C

PO_2	sat of Hb	dissolved O_2 ml/100ml
10	13.5	0.03
20	35.0	0.06
30	57.0	0.09
40	75.0	0.12
50	83.5	0.15
60	89.0	0.18
70	92.7	0.21
80	94.5	0.24
90	96.5	0.27
100	97.4	0.30

PER CENT SATURATION OF HAEMOGLOBIN

PO_2 (mm Hg)

Figure 2

105

because although there may be little threat to life, the integrity of suture lines may be threatened by arterial desaturation.

Post-traumatic Pulmonary Insufficiency

Increasing numbers of patients are being encountered who after major surgery or major injury show a respiratory insufficiency syndrome characterised by stiff lungs, progressive hypoxia, and the chest X-ray appearances of diffuse consolidation which is usually maximal at the hila. Many of the causes of this problem are preventable: over-transfusion or over-infusion (a frequent culprit) by careful attention to the management of shock and to the fluid balance chart; aspiration of irritant vomitus, by keeping the stomach empty with a nasogastric tube or by gastrostomy; oxygen toxicity, by avoiding inspired concentrations in excess of 30%. The most difficult factors to prevent are those leading to micro-embolisation of the pulmonary blood vessels. This occurs in two main circumstances: *platelet-fibrin aggregates* from massive transfusion of stored blood; and *fat* embolisation usually after long bone fractures. Reasonable precautions are as follows:

1. Whenever more than 4 units of blood are to be transfused a *dacron mesh filter* should be incorporated in the giving line.

2. Fat embolus should be suspected if a patient develops tachypnoea, drowsiness, or skin petechiae in the first few days after injury. You may look for fat globules in the retina (rare) and in the urine (uncommon) but be sure to determine *arterial* pO_2 and do a *chest X-ray* both of which often show more dramatic changes than would be expected from the patient's appearance. There is no specific treatment for fat embolus and the course of pulmonary insufficiency from this cause tends to be unrelenting. It is important to be prepared to start positive pressure ventilation early before the lungs become irretrievably stiff.

Acute Postoperative Mental Disturbances

We have already mentioned that patients admitted for surgical treatment may be under severe stress and thus behave differently from normal. Sometimes an acute mental disturbance is found in the perioperative period, more usually after operation. When this occurs it is vital to sort out in a logical manner those things that are likely to be the result of an emotional upset and those which are related to physiological or pathological events. In particular it is *never* safe to label a patient as 'mad' or 'having the DT's' just because preoperatively he was known to be a little odd or dependent on alcohol. There are many things such as hypoxia, electrolyte imbalance, and severe sepsis, that can mimic delirium tremens in particular and which if not treated early and precisely can lead to the patient's death. The best approach is to run through the following list of causes which is arranged according to frequency and priority in management. If, and only if, no cause is found having gone through this routine is it then justifiable to label the patient as having an acute primary mental disturbance such as a psychosis, and then only after consultation with an enlightened psychiatrist.

1. **Hypoxia.** Obtain and rapidly analyse an arterial blood gas sample. A pAO_2 of less than 50 mm Hg should be treated urgently.

2. **Metabolic disturbance.** Hyper and hypoglycaemia (ward check using a glucose meter); low serum sodium concentration (do electrolyte values); very low or very high serum calcium concentration; low scrum magnesium concentration (think of both according to the history and check subsequently).

3. **Sepsis.** Generalised sepsis—syn. septicaemia—(draw blood for culture but institute treatment).

4. **Intracranial disorders.** Head injury (fall before operation). Cerebral oedema (over infusion).

5. **Situational disorders.** Sleep lack; sensory barrage; inappropriate drugs (check the prescription sheet).

6. **Alcohol.** Delirium tremens (from history of alcohol intake).

Do not make the diagnosis of the last until all others have been excluded. It is one of the least common causes.

The treatment of delirium tremens has become much simpler since the introduction of chlormethiazole (heminevrin). It is given as an 0.8% solution initially in an adult at a rate of 5–10 mls per minute. Individual responses vary considerably and it is essential that the patient is carefully observed because he can quickly lapse into deep coma.

Low Blood Pressure States

It is often difficult to determine the precise cause of a low blood pressure state, but to do this is of the very greatest importance to the survival of the patient. You must first check that the blood pressure is indeed low: make sure that the sphygmomanometer cuff is properly placed, check auscultatory readings by palpation, try the other arm.

The three major causes of low blood pressure states are:

1. **Reduced blood volume, low cardiac output** = surgical shock. Pallor, sweating, cool extremities, tachycardia, narrow pulse pressure. Consider the possibility of occult bleeding, or pre-existing Na^+ and water depletion. The usual explanation is inadequate replacement of blood previously lost or continuing haemorrhage.

2. **Normal blood volume, normal to high cardiac output** = widespread arteriolar dilation. This may occur:
   (a) as a consequence of general or regional anaesthesia; of premedicant drugs such as triflupromazine; or of the more specific vasodilator drugs designed to produce hypotension. The patient looks and feels well, and the condition is usually benign: in most instances no more than careful supervision is necessary.
   (b) As a pre-terminal stage of surgical shock, despite apparently adequate blood-volume replacement; as a result of overwhelming infection (particularly with gram -ve organisms); of the liberation or introduction of gram -ve endotoxins; rarely of genuine adrenal failure. The patient is obviously gravely ill and desperate measures are called for. On the whole it is probably wiser and more profitable to *overtransfuse* with plasma or blood, than to use *vasoconstrictor agents*. Intravenous *hydrocortisone* (250–500 mg) or *prednisone* (50–100 mg) is sometimes dramatically successful, but as a pharmacological agent rather than because of 'adrenal exhaustion'. Where overwhelming infection is suspected, intravenous gentamicin 100 mg or kanamycin 500 mg are probably the most useful antibiotics.

3. **Normal to increased blood volume, low cardiac output** = heart failure—congestive, or specifically right or left-sided. The signs of these conditions should be sought, and the cause: dysrhythmia of sudden onset; pulmonary embolisation; myocardial infarction; K^+ intoxication or gross K^+ depletion; gram -ve septicaemia. *ECG evidence of myocardial infarction should not be too readily accepted*—it is a rare complication in the immediate postoperative period, and the

ECG changes may be a result of, rather than a cause of, the low blood pressure.

'Sick cell' Hyponatraemia

Some seriously ill, frequently malnourished and not uncommonly septic, patients show a paradoxical picture of low serum sodium concentration and moderatly elevated serum potassium concentration. These patients lack energy to drive the sodium pump and need glucose and insulin. Carefully controlled therapy with hourly intravenous boluses of 50% dextrose with added soluble insulin at 120 u/l and potassium 40 mmol/1 is used. Initially plasma potassium, sodium and glucose concentrations are measured every 2 hours until stable levels of glucose (5.5–10.5 mmol/1 and potassium 4–5 mmol/1) are reached. Thereafter 8 hourly measurements suffice.

Deep Vein Thrombosis

Prospective studies by phlebography or gamma detection of ^{125}I-fibrinogen deposition have shown a 30% incidence of *deep calf vein thrombosis* in middle-aged patients undergoing operation. The incidence of *ilio femoral vein thrombosis* is still unknown. There has thus been emphasis on double-blind trials of prophylaxis against calf vein thrombosis. Conventional early postoperative ambulation, elastic stockings or bandages, lower limb elevation and physiotherapy are ineffective. The following regimens have been shown to be statistically effective:

Heparin—Calcium heparin s.c.i. 5000 i.u. 2 hours pre op., 24 hours post op., then 12 hourly for 5 days.

Dextran 70—1 litre 6% in 0.85% NaCl given over 6 hours, commencing on induction of anaesthesia.

Calf muscles—Peroperative square-wave stimulation, intermittent compression, or passive exercise.
N.B.: *None of the above has yet been shown conclusively to prevent the potentially lethal ilio-femoral vein thrombosis, or to prevent pulmonary embolism. At the time of writing there is a trend away from*

preventive measures based on modifying coagulation (heparin and dextran).

With a real incidence of calf vein thrombosis of 30%, undetectable in most patients by clinical means, there is no longer point in routine daily examination of the legs. Nevertheless *low grade fever*, palpable localised *calf tenderness*, or uni- or bi-lateral ankle *oedema* with increased depth of skin colour or bluish hue, creates a high index of suspicion of major deep vein thrombosis. Before potentially dangerous therapy is instituted, objective proof *must* be obtained by phlebography.

The best method of treating deep vein thrombosis is in doubt. A conventional approach is:

1. If signs are confined to the calf, and either Doppler flowmetry or phlebography shows the thrombus is confined to leg veins, prescribe continuing activity with a firm below knee elastic bandage.

2. If signs are extending or thrombus is detected in the iliofemoral veins by Doppler flowmetry or phlebography, use the same treatment schedule as for pulmonary embolus (see later). Venous thrombectomy in this circumstance has usually not prevented emboli, nor left the patient with a patent vein.

Pulmonary Embolisation

Prospective perfusion/ventilation scanning has shown an 8% incidence of pulmonary embolus in middle-aged surgical patients. The clinically recognised incidence is about 0.5%. There have been no adequately conducted trials that show prophylactic therapy to be effective in reducing the incidence.

The following should create a high index of suspicion that a patient has suffered a moderate sized (e.g. lobar) pulmonary embolus: *breathlessness, pleurisy* (with or without pleural rub), or *haemoptysis*. The following suggest a large pulmonary embolus (blocking at least one main pulmonary artery): *severe breathlessness, faintness, collapse with hypotension, R ventricular heave, gallop rhythm, split pulmonary second sound, elevated R atrial* (jugular venous) *pressure*. Before potentially dangerous therapy is instituted (or continued), objective proof is desirable by *lung perfusion scanning* or by *pulmonary angiography*. Electrocardiographic signs are unreliable, often dangerously so.

The choices of immediate therapy are:

110

1. *Pulmonary embolectomy* is rarely indicated, requires cardiopulmonary bypass, and demands absolute proof of diagnosis by pulmonary angiography.

2. Fibrinolytic therapy by *streptokinase* or *urokinase* for 24–36 hours followed by heparization for at least 7 days. *This is not applicable within 10–14 days of operation*. It is otherwise the most effective therapy (though requiring excellent laboratory control and with significant risk of bleeding episodes).

3. *Anticoagulant therapy*. This in practice means intravenous *heparin*. 10000 i.u. IV stat., then about 1000 i.u./hour to maintain clotting time at 10–15 min; or better, to maintain the activated partial thromboplastin time, kaolincephalin clotting time, or thrombin clotting time within the limits recommended by your laboratory.

4. When a *low cardiac output state* is present, and is either immediately life-threatening or does not respond to above therapy, give isoprenaline 2–4 μg/min, and oxygen by face mask or endotracheal tube.

5. When there is proven *recurrence* of pulmonary embolus during or after the above forms of therapy, *inferior vena caval interruption* by ligation, plication, serrated clip, or caval 'umbrella' may be undertaken.

A flow-chart, summarising this information, is on p. 112.

Longer-term therapy, after the initial or recurrent episode has been controlled, is predicated by the risk of continuing pulmonary embolisation. This in turn is dictated by the presence and anatomical location (size) of deep vein thrombi. We therefore recommend that every patient who has sustained a pulmonary embolus should undergo *bilateral lower limb phlebography*. If thrombus is detected in the popliteal vein or more proximally we suggest that a 10–14 day course of heparin therapy be followed by a 6 week to 6 month course of oral prothrombin-depressant therapy (phenindione, warfarin).

Intestinal Obstruction and Nasogastric Decompression

A better understanding of the physiology of the gut after operation has reduced the need for pre- and postoperative decompression by nasogastric tube or gastrostomy. It appears that after uncomplicated procedures intestinal motility returns rapidly if somewhat unevenly, so that the small bowel is propulsive again within 24 hours. However,

111

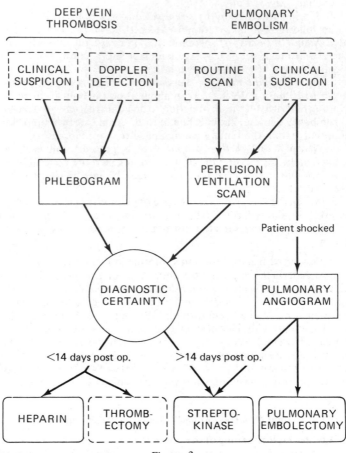

DEEP VEIN
THROMBOSIS

PULMONARY
EMBOLISM

CLINICAL
SUSPICION

DOPPLER
DETECTION

ROUTINE
SCAN

CLINICAL
SUSPICION

PHLEBOGRAM

PERFUSION
VENTILATION
SCAN

Patient shocked

DIAGNOSTIC
CERTAINTY

PULMONARY
ANGIOGRAM

<14 days post op.

>14 days post op.

HEPARIN

THROMB-
ECTOMY

STREPTO-
KINASE

PULMONARY
EMBOLECTOMY

Figure 3

112

if the stomach has been vagally denervated or has an anastomosis or suture line at its distal end it may not effectively empty itself for at least 48 hours. The colon is likewise sluggish in that though it is not adynamic it appears not to regain fully effective and coordinated contractions for about the same length of time. These disturbances can usually be handled merely by withholding oral liquids for 24–36 hours. If this is done and there is still doubt about the stomach being able to empty, the matter can be settled by the following simple technique which avoids the risk of putting liquids into an atonic stomach:

1. Take a preliminary portable supine film of the abdomen if contrast medium has been used to investigate the gastrointestinal tract in the immediate past.

2. Administer 50 ml of water soluble contrast medium (gastrografin).

3. Lay the patient slightly to the right, and propped up so that the medium does not pool in the fundus, for 1 hour.

4. Take a further film at the end of 1 hour. Normal progress is indicated by seeing contrast medium in the distal small bowel. Do not expect this technique to give effective anatomical detail; however, with the radiologist's cooperation it can occasionally be used to search for a leak in a gastrointestinal or oesophageal suture line.

A similar procedure is in order when after an abdominal operation a patient vomits for a reason that is not obvious. If the contrast medium progresses normally consider causes outside the gastrointestinal tract, such as idiosyncrasy to drugs. Use of this procedure may save the unnecessary and unpleasant passage of a nasogastric tube.

Preoperative nasogastric tubes

In *elective surgery* there is rarely a need for a preoperative tube. If one is thought likely to be needed either pre- or postoperatively it can be inserted on the operating table.

In emergency surgery it is often thought desirable to empty the stomach before anaesthesia is induced. However, bear in mind two things: that semisolid food or clotted blood cannot pass through an oesophageal tube; that attempts to pass a tube in a sick patient (particularly in shock) may initiate retching and vomiting which defeat the object of the exercise, and may even lead to aspiration into the respiratory tree. The conclusion is simple: either do not pass tube at all and cooperate personally with the anaesthetist in applying cricoid pressure, or abandon attempts at the first sign of difficulty.

Technique of cricoid pressure. The supine patient is asked to swallow and then to extend the head so that the oesophagus is stretched on the spine and is thus less likely to slip away when pressure is applied. The fingers then press back firmly on the cricoid cartilage as the anaesthetist induces anaesthesia and passes the endotracheal tube. Pressure must be unrelenting until the cuff is inflated and there is no doubt whatever that it is the trachea that has been intubated. Do not apply cricoid pressure if the patient is retching—oesophageal rupture may result.

Postoperative nasogastric tubes

Each surgeon will have his own routine (showing incidentally that no one as yet has all the answers). As implied already many patients do not need intubation at all, others only for a very short time. If the operation has been complicated by peritoneal contamination or by an extensive dissection, decompression may be required for many days. The choice then lies between *nasogastric intubation*, and *gastrostomy* done at the time of operation. The former is associated with more respiratory complications, the latter with an increased risk of abdominal wall sepsis. Both are managed by

1. Continuous drainage.
2. Supplementary syringe aspiration at 1–2 hourly intervals.
3. Nil by mouth (except ice chips to suck) in order to avoid complexities of water and electrolyte arithmetic.

If a gastrostomy has been fashioned, the tube should not be removed in less than eight days to minimise the slight risk of leakage at the seal between abdominal wall and the anterior aspect of the stomach.

Temperature Charts and their Interpretation

Most surgeons, and particularly house surgeons, spend a great deal of time looking at temperature charts, yet surprisingly little thought

114

has gone into their analysis. The subject is still in its infancy, but in the repetitive situation of surgery we can distinguish five broad patterns which, while not absolutely diagnostic, are nevertheless strongly suspicious of particular events (see Figure 4).

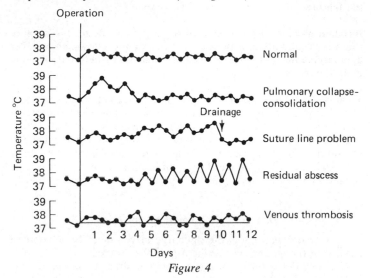

Figure 4

Normal. Even after quite major surgery, provided tissue damage is slight and traumatised tissue is not left in situ, oral temperature rise is small. Two or three readings in the range 37.8–38° over a period of 24 hours is all that should be expected.

Postoperative pulmonary collapse-consolidation with possible super-added infection. This event takes place within an hour or two of leaving the operating table. The effect of retained secretions is an early marked rise in oral temperature to 38.5–38.8°C. Provided that physiotherapy is good and the sputum block eliminated, the fever subsides within 48–72 hours by lysis and the afebrile chart of normal convalescence is resumed.

Suture line dehiscence. It is probable that most suture line problems are the consequence of ischaemia. Therefore as might be expected

115

they begin to manifest themselves at 48–72 hours with a low grade fever which is accumulative over the next approximately four to five days. If a drain has been led down to the site of anastomosis then disruption may be followed by fistula formation and lysis. Otherwise the features of a residual abscess supervene.

Residual abscess. If pus is spilt or organisms introduced at surgery there is usually a latent period before systemic signs such as fever begin to manifest themselves. 72 hours may go by before a swinging fever develops.

Venous thrombosis when it is spreading is accompanied quite frequently by fever. In that many thromboses begin on the operating table the low grade fever which characterises the condition (36.8–37.8°C) may occur at any time after operation. The diagnosis should be strongly suspected if such a fever persists for 48 hours or more without signs of another complication such as suture line breakdown.

Disruption of Abdominal Incisions

1. An early warning is the discharge of yellow or blood-stained fluid from the wound, indicating a peritoneal defect.

2. Delay in the return of bowel function after abdominal operations is occasionally but rarely due to a gap in the peritoneal suture, allowing a coil of bowel to enter the wound.

3. The skin may gape when sutures cut out or are removed—and there may be underlying deeper disruption not at first obvious.

In all these circumstances the incision is explored and resutured as soon as possible. Inform your senior at once when suspicion arises (before secondary infection has occurred).

Where bowel is visible through a disrupted wound, cover it with a sterile sheet soaked in intravenous saline (NOT cottonwool or similar material), give a sedative premedication, inform your senior and warn the operating theatre and an anaesthetist.

Disrupted wounds can usually be closed only by the use of through-and-through sutures, which should be left in place for at least 14 days. A further episode of frank wound disruption is uncommon (but not unknown): after a first episode consideration should be given to providing supplementary intravenous alimentation (see p. 96) if healing-failure can be attributed to malnutrition. After wound disruption there is a greatly increased incidence of incisional hernia.

Paralytic (Adynamic) Ileus

1. In its true form (complete small and large bowel paralysis with no source of mechanical obstruction), the condition is rare. Some causes are: *widespread peritonitis* (perforated hollow viscus), *retroperitoneal haemorrhage*, *metabolic disturbance* (uraemia, hypokalaemia, hypercalcaemia), *neurologic abnormality* (quadriplegia), *immobility* (plaster bed, curare paralysis), *drugs* (ganglion-blocking, antidepressant).
2. Management of the true form includes:
    (a) Correction of the precipitating disturbance if possible
    (b) Nasogastric suction, IV fluids, and wait patiently
    (c) When patience is exhausted, try pharmacologic manipulation with sympathetic blockade (e.g. guanethidine IV 1 mg/min up to 10 mg), followed by cholinergic stimulation (e.g. bethanechol 0.5 mg IM/min up to 5 mg, or prostigmine 0.1 mg IM/min up to 1 mg). The administration of guanethidine must be done with the patient lying flat and with an arterial blood pressure recording every five minutes.

Post-traumatic Gastroduodenal Haemorrhage

It is fortunately fairly rare now for a patient to experience a massive upper gastrointestinal haemorrhage as a consequence of what is generally called a 'stress ulcer' or 'ulcer'. The major determinant is sepsis following in the wake of an acute injury or surgical procedure. The technical management of the incident, if it is allowed to occur, is much as for any other instance of upper gastrointestinal bleeding (p. 139). However, prevention is better than cure. High risk groups include:

1. Major surgery with or followed by sepsis as already indicated.
2. Ruptured aortic aneurysm.
3. Burns.

4. Severe head injuries.

5. Massive small bowel resection.

6. Rarely, perforated or bleeding peptic ulcer in which Zollinger–Ellison syndrome (p. 142) is suspected.

Two methods of prophylaxis are possible:

1. If the gastrointestinal tract is intact and functioning alkalis may be used but have to be in large doses, e.g. 200–300 ml aluminium hydroxide daily in divided doses, or continuously down a nasogastric tube.

2. In other circumstances cimetidine 1 g daily by continuous intravenous infusion.

The need for such energetic prophylaxis is far from firmly established except in sepsis.

12. SURGICAL EMERGENCIES

There are not many situations where seconds or minutes may save or lose a life. Some of these are discussed below. Individually they occur rarely, but one or other may crop up every few months.

Cardiac Arrest

It is vital that you familiarise yourself with the instructions regarding the procedure in this situation, which should be posted in every ward and operating theatre, together with an appropriate emergency kit. Similarly, before carrying out any operation, however minor, under general or local anaesthesia you **MUST** be prepared and able to carry out intermittent cardiac compression.

Additional points worth remembering are:

1. A *single* sharp blow to the precordium may sometimes restore heart action when it is in standstill.

2. In the operating theatre, *open-chest cardiac pumping* may still be the best way of re-establishing and maintaining an adequate cardiac output. Outside the operating theatre *closed-chest sternal compression* is the best management.

3. Before undertaking either technique, there must be present an

assistant who can provide *adequate pulmonary ventilation*. This is doubly important in that the commonest cause of cardiac standstill or fibrillation in surgical practice is anoxia.

4. *Adequate cardiac pumping* (as judged by a palpable carotid or femoral pulse), with adequate ventilation, will keep the patient alive. **NOW** call for expert help, which may include **ECG** monitoring, electrical defibrillation, drugs and cardiac pacing.

5. When cardiac arrest occurs in a dying patient, where the primary disease is incurable, or where cardiac arrest occurs as part of some grave illness not rapidly reversible, cardiac resuscitation is pointless.

Tension Pneumothorax

This may occur spontaneously but in the surgical context it is tension pneumothorax following chest injury which is of greatest concern. It is vital to recognise it *clinically* by the gross tracheal and cardiac displacement and evidence of substantial pneumothorax (breath sounds may sometimes be audible through a pneumothorax). You should immediately call the surgeon or registrar and obtain the emergency equipment for inserting an underwater seal drain. Nowadays the underwater seal drain equipment usually takes the form of a disposable set, consisting of a wide bore needle surrounded by a catheter. After infiltrating the skin and chest wall down to the pleura with local anaesthetic, a nick is made in the skin with a scalpel blade, the catheter and needle inserted into the pleural cavity, the needle withdrawn and the catheter connected to an underwater seal drain (or, as a temporary measure, to a one-way valve). The preferred sites for insertion of the catheter are the 4th or 5th intercostal space in the mid-axillary line, or the 2nd interspace anteriorly.

If the patient's condition is *rapidly deteriorating* immediate decompression of the pleural cavity must be performed by inserting a wide bore needle, even in the temporary absence of tubing and drainage bottle. If there seems time, inject local anaesthetic into the proposed site of insertion and accompany the patient *personally* to the X-ray department for an *urgent chest X-ray*, taking with you the equipment for insertion of the underwater drain. N.B. This is one respiratory emergency where *endotracheal intubation* is valueless as an isolated procedure.

A particularly dangerous form of tension pneumothorax is that which occurs during general anaesthesia. Positive pressure ventila tion will convert any pneumothorax into the life-threatening tension form. In the anaesthetised, ventilated patient, the only manifestations may be a fall in blood pressure and cyanosis, the cause of which may not be immediately apparent. It is mandatory therefore that, in any patient with a pneumothorax, an underwater seal drain is inserted before the induction of anaesthesia.

Extra-dural Haemorrhage
(See also Chapter 28)

Where there is a rapid progression of signs suggesting this condition in a patient with a head injury you should:

1. Ensure the patient has an adequate airway and there are facilities for artificial ventilation (at least a double-ended airway).
2. Notify the neurosurgeon on call and/or the surgeon in charge of the patient.
3. Alert the neurosurgical theatre staff, if asked to do so.
4. Alert the anaesthetist on call.
5. Make sure facilities for a head shave are available.
6. Take blood for urgent crossmatching of 2 units.

External Haemorrhage from a Major Artery

It is scarcely necessary to say that the bleeding should be controlled by continued direct pressure, using a hand and swab, and that *you personally* should continue with this until help arrives.

Respiratory Obstruction

This may be due to many causes, e.g.

1. **Coma** In an unconscious or semi-conscious patient the commonest cause of respiratory obstruction is the *tongue*. Such a patient should be nursed on his side, with the head extended and the jaw forward.
2. **After operation** on head and neck, due to haematoma formation. If obstruction seems severe and of rapid onset, and there is evidence of substantial haematoma, the wound should be reopened in the ward. This is very rarely necessary.

3. **Trauma:**
(a) *Jaw fractures* and soft tissue injuries—insertion of the finger into the mouth and traction to bring the jaw forward may relieve. Beware the *broken denture* as an obstructing agent.
(b) *Neck laceration* involving trachea, as in suicidal cut throat. The tracheal fistula can usually be employed as an adequate temporary airway.

4. **Foreign body impacted in larynx.** This is one of the rare situations where if a largyngoscope and the necessary skill to use it are not *immediately* available, *immediate tracheostomy* may save life.

Where upper respiratory obstruction is increasing, and where the local circumstances permit, *endotracheal intubation* should be carried out. If the cause of the obstruction does not permit this, at once personally take the patient to the *operating theatre*, while administering high flow oxygen via a face mask. If possible, have an assistant ring theatre to prepare for urgent tracheostomy, and alert your senior.

Accident Victims and the Seriously Ill

One of the recurring problems with severely ill or accident patients is ordering priorities so that the important things for immediate management and thus survival are done *at once*. There is always a tendency for X-rays to be done because of their possible future medicolegal significance or because the Casualty Officer quite rightly does not want to be castigated for missing something, when what the patient needs is urgent transfer to the operating theatre for control of bleeding. Nursing and administrative staff may become preoccupied with getting details of little significance about the patient or carrying out routine matters such as washing and undressing, when what he needs is urgent resuscitation, anaesthesia, and definitive treatment of the wounds. Constant thought and attention is needed by all (not least the houseman) to make sure that everyone is continually and constructively busy in the way most suited to the patient's most important problems. We are not suggesting that corners be cut, only that a realistic analysis is made of priorities. As a guide consider the following list*:

* From Hamilton Bailey's Emergency Surgery Ed. H. A. F. Dudley, John Wright, Bristol, 1977.

Immediate priority

Airway.

Mechanics of respiration.

Restoration of blood volume and arrest of massive bleeding.

Urgent

Relief of cerebral compression by craniotomy.

Assisted respiration if relief of obstruction and/or correction of embarrassed mechanisms has proved ineffective.

High priority

Relief of severe pain by administering a narcotic analgesic (p. 20, but not without consultation in patient with head injury, respiratory inadequacy or hypovolaemia).

Laparotomy and less commonly thoracotomy for internal injuries (on occasion this may be required more urgently to establish the conditions under which resuscitation may proceed).

Exploration of damaged major blood vessels and/or expanding haematoma.

Exploration of pelvis for injuries to bladder, urethra, female genitalia.

Relief of constricting limb burns.

Decompression of fascial compartments.

Fixation of fractures if highly unstable or associated with blood vessel or nerve injury.

Less urgent

Fractures of long bones without the above (however, if there is a call for anaesthesia for other reasons the fractures should if possible be definitively treated at the same time).

Minimal priority

Minor fractures of limbs or trunk, minor lacerations and small burns.

13. SURGICAL INFECTIONS

General

Two large groups of infected cases are met with in surgical wards:
where the infection is the *primary* cause of admission,
or, where the infection is *acquired in hospital*.

A great deal of attention is being paid to the problem of infection and cross-infection. It is quite disastrous when a patient acquires a significant wound or other infection which occurs only because he *is* in hospital. There are certain rules with regard to the management of those with infections:

1. *All* patients with an infection capable of being disseminated, whether this be a discharging abscess or wound, gross pulmonary or urinary tract sepsis, or open, infected, skin lesions such as chronic leg ulcers or bed sores, MUST be isolated, either in a sideroom of the ward or better in an isolation block. These precautions are especially important if the patient is receiving or has received an *antibiotic*.

2. Material from the lesion must be sent for bacteriological culture in all cases.

Antibiotics
(See also Chapter 6 p. 57)

As you will soon discover, these are used sparingly in surgery. The reasons are:

1. Most staphylococcal infections may be presumed to be resistant to the commoner and safer antibiotics.

2. Most infections in surgical wards present no danger to life and will be controlled more readily and effectively by adequate surgery than by antibiotics.

3. Therefore, in the majority of cases antibiotics are not used at all, and certainly not before the organism has been cultured and the in vitro sensitivity determined.

4. There are however certain important exceptions to this rule, when it is very important to use antibiotics, though if possible not until material has been sent for culture. Those exceptions are *spreading infections* such as septicaemia, peritonitis, pneumonia, and where there is risk of, or actual, infection with *anaerobic organisms* such as Cl. tetani or gas-forming bacteria.

Gram-negative Septicaemia

This has replaced infections with *Staph. pyogenes* as the commonest life-threatening infection in surgical patients.

1. The *microorganisms* are usually, in order of frequency, *E. coli; Aerobacter aerogenes; Ps. aeruginosa; Proteus; Bacteroides*.

2. The *clinical circumstances* are, again in approximate order of frequency, urinary tract manipulation (catheterisation, cytoscopy, prostatic biopsy); biliary tract disease or manipulation (cholangitis, exploration common bile duct); burns; severe peritonitis; prolonged IV infusion.

3. The *manifestations* are:
   (a) **Mild**—fever, rigors, warm hypotension
   (b) **Severe**—fever, rigors, disorientation, hyperventilation, cold hypotension, metabolic acidosis.

In the mild form the patient is normovolaemic and survival rate is high. In the severe form the patient usually has a complex pre-existing surgical condition, is hypovolaemic and the survival rate is low.

4. *Management*. In all but the very mildest and transient episodes it is essential to do the following:
   (a) Draw blood for culture at least twice daily until at least two cultures have been reported negative.
   (b) Establish a central venous line (p. 82) and control replacement with crystalloid or colloid by measuring CVP. Considerable volumes may be needed in, for example, peritonitis. A level of 9 cm of water should be aimed for.
   (c) Call for urgent help from experts such as interested surgeons, anaesthetists and cardiologists and, if possible, transfer the patient to an intensive care unit.
   (d) Have an electrocardiogram so as to be sure that you are not confusing septicaemia with myocardial infarction.
   (e) Establish whether the patient is or is not acidotic by arterial pH measurement. Correct acidosis if present (p. 91).
   (f) Administer a 'best guess' antibiotic or combination of antibiotics, preferably after consultation with your senior and/or the microbiologist.
   (g) In patients who make a poor response to volume loading consider an intravenous bolus of methyl prednisolone 40 mgm. Failure to respond is common and it is useless to repeat the dose.

(h) Inotropic agents, such as dopamine, are sometimes indicated, but see (c) above.

Abscesses

The principles of treatment of these are as follows:

1. With rare exceptions, whatever the situation, when there is pus it must be let out. Antibiotics will partly or completely sterilise an abscess, but will rarely cure it or the patient. Conversely, adequate drainage renders an antibiotic unnecessary.

2. In certain instances *fluctuation*, the classical sign of an abscess, *appears late* due to the quality of the surrounding tissues, e.g. breast, hand, foot and digits, parotid, ischio-rectal fossa. In these cases, if there has been inflammation for more than 48 hours, pus may be presumed to be present and the part should be explored forthwith.

3. An abscess should *never* be opened under local anaesthesia, if only because exploration is limited. A regional block is sometimes acceptable.

4. In opening any abscess the incision must provide adequate *drainage* and the abscess cavity must be *explored* to break down loculi and remove all dead tissue.

5. A swab of the pus must *always* be sent to the laboratory for culture during the day, or be personally plated-out at night.

6. In any unusual abscess part of the wall should be sent for *histological examination*, and thought given to Tb or fungal culture.

Wound Infections

These may be present in several forms usually with accompanying **pain**:

1. **Superficial reddening** of skin margins ('stitch abscesses'). These require no specific treatment.

2. **Abscess formation.**
   (a) *Subcutaneous*—removal of stitches and/or probing of wound is sufficient.
   (b) *Deep* in the wound or intraperitoneal—formal drainage may be necessary *when the abscess points*. If non-absorbable sutures have been implanted, they may have to be removed.

3. **Spreading infection**, often streptococcal, sometimes anaerobic. Antibiotics are invaluable.

125

4. After *cardiovascular surgery* a wound infection may be lethal because of secondary haemorrhage. Here massive doses of an antibiotic which is active against the 'hospital' staphylococcus may be vital.

Urinary Tract Infections

Primary. Infections can either involve the bladder (cystitis) or bladder and renal parenchyma (pyelonephritis). Whilst bladder infections are symptomatically distressing, it is infections of the renal parenchyma that cause scarring and impaired renal function. The tendency is to treat initial infections with only short courses of antibiotics (24–48 hr). This approach appears to have two advantages: first, it will cure the majority of infections and reduce antibiotic consumption and, second, if the infection persists, it suggests that there is some underlying abnormality and further investigation is warranted.

Secondary (see section on prostatectomy).

14. ABDOMINAL PAIN

A high proportion of patients sent into hospital with the provisional diagnosis of acute appendicitis have insufficient symptoms and signs of this disease to warrant operation. In the absence of a positive alternative diagnosis they are therefore treated by bed rest and either IV or oral fluids until the abdominal pain or fever has subsided.

In most cases no positive diagnosis will be reached. Investigate all such patients by:

1. Haematocrit, WBC count and film
2. PA chest X-ray
3. Microscopic examination of urine.

Some of the causes of abdominal pain for which patients may be sent to a surgical ward as having appendicitis are:

Virus and related infections, especially in children, of a wide variety: non-specific respiratory and entero-viruses, hepatitis, poliomyelitis, infective mononucleosis, measles, mumps. When appendicitis seems

126

unlikely it is worthwhile enquiring for prodromal or associated symptoms of these diseases.

Ectopic pregnancy

Salpingitis

Right-sided urinary tract lesions.

Biliary tract lesions

Pneumonia.

Intestinal obstruction, especially intussusception.

Perforation of a duodenal ulcer with minimal leakage down the right paracolic gutter.

Pancreatitis

Acute arthritis R. hip

Herpes zoster

Numerous miscellaneous conditions: diabetic ketosis, myocardial infarction, diaphragmatic pleurisy, Bornholm disease, spinal root lesion, collagen disease, acute haemolytic episodes, lead poisoning, and acute porphyria, to name but a few. Many of these conditions are rare, but collectively they are not uncommon. They may require other special investigations.

'Mesenteric adenitis' correctly defines a pathological state but is not a diagnosis—it *may* be caused by one of the lymphoid reticuloses or a virus, more commonly the latter.

Young adults with ureteric colic which has unusual features *may* suffer from drug addiction or a psychological disorder.

While abdominal pain is frequently associated with psychological disturbance, this common combination does not exclude organic abdominal disease. If a gynaecological cause is suspected, an examination under anaesthesia or a laparoscopy using local or general anaesthesia, may be undertaken.

15. APPENDICITIS

History

The important points to record are:

1. When the pain started.
2. Where it started.
3. Where it is now.
4. Has there been loss of appetite, nausea or vomiting?
5. Recent bowel habit—frequency and nature of bowel motions from 24 hours before onset of pain.
6. Has there been urinary frequency?
7. Is there a history of a previous similar attack?

Examination

Record:

1. The exact site of maximal abdominal tenderness and guarding (percussion may help to localise).
2. The presence or absence of a mass.
3. The presence or absence of rectal tenderness.

Investigations

No special investigations are necessary when there is no doubt about the diagnosis and the patient is young. In the patient who is not operated on, or in whom the appendix is found to be normal, *it is important to obtain investigations as for abdominal pain.*

Complications

Peritonitis

If *general peritonitis* is obvious or suspected, start antibiotics parenterally with the premedication. Three regimens are currently in common use—

> metronidazole + cephalosporin (e.g. cefoxitin)
> lincomycin + gentamicin
> lincomycin + cefoxitin

If *general peritonitis* is found at operation, start antibiotic immediately.

If *significant local peritonitis* is found at operation, antibiotic may be of value.

Abscesses

In most cases *fever* will subside over 2–5 days. If it persists or recurs, suspect:

1. *Abscess in or deep to wound*—look for reddening, undue tenderness or induration of wound.
2. *Pelvic abscess*—perform a rectal examination.
3. *Subphrenic abscess*—examine lung bases, chest X-ray.

With the exception of subphrenic abscess, the remainder will either:
Discharge through the wound, or
Discharge into bowel—usually caecum or rectum—or vagina.

Vomiting

If this occurs more than 12 hours after operation it suggests a *small bowel obstruction* on the basis of inflammatory oedema or local or adynamic *ileus*.

Look for *abdominal distension*, *general guarding*, absent or obstructive bowel sounds, persistent or increasing *fever* or *tachycardia*. Plain X-ray of abdomen is advisable. *When in doubt*, start gastric aspiration, set up IV drip, and notify your senior.

Late obstruction

Small bowel obstruction may occur later than the 8th day, due to an *abscess* (fever) or to fibro-fibrinous *adhesions* (no fever). In the latter instance operation is usually the safest course.

16. ARTERIAL SURGERY

Limbs
(See also p. 134)

Investigation of patients suspected of this disorder aims at answering in sequence these questions:

1. Is there an *arterial block or stenosis*?
2. *Where* is the block?
3. Are symptoms severe enough, with respect to *pain*, *work* or *limb survival*, to suggest direct arterial surgery?
4. Does the patient's *general condition* admit of direct surgery, with respect to:
   (a) Coronary disease.
   (b) Cerebrovascular disease.
   (c) Pulmonary disease.
   (d) Renal disease.
   (e) Diabetes mellitus.
5. Is the local arterial condition *technically* amenable to direct surgery?

History

1. *Leg symptoms*—
   claudication and walking distance at onset
   rest pain or numbness in the foot
   gangrene
2. *Time relation* of onset of these symptoms.
3. *Site of claudication*—
   foot
   calf
   thigh
   buttock
4. Failure of erection.
5. Is the patient incapacitated by his leg symptoms?
6. Symptomatic evidence of disorders affecting his general condition.

Examination

1. *Gangrene* or *foot ulceration*, colour or wasting of limb.
2. Unilateral *skin coldness* of limb and its *upper limit*.
3. *Pulses*—these are most important and must be accurately recorded, as present (+), absent (−), or diminished (±).
4. *Bruits*—listen at carotid bifurcations, *aortic bifurcation* and over *femoral arteries*.
N.B. If a bruit is heard, check that it does not come from *aortic valve* or *aortic coarctation*.
5. Record *blood pressure* in both upper limbs.

General investigations

Haematology screen, including platelets
Biochemical screen, including blood urea and blood glucose
Plasma lipids
Serology for syphilis
   If a 'collagen' disease is suspected, add:
   ESR
   Serum protein electrophoresis
   Cold agglutininins, cryoproteins
   Anti-nuclear antibody (or LE cells).
ECG
Chest X-ray

Special investigations

These depend on the policy and facilities of the unit, but may include indirect measurement of blood pressure at the ankles and direct measurement of femoral artery pressures.

Arteriogram

This is the *last* investigation to be undertaken, if the patient has not already been excluded from surgery. Specify the arteries about which information is sought, and the route suggested by the surgeon for arterial puncture (e.g. 'via Right femoral', etc.).

Internal Carotid Atherosclerosis

History

1. Precise history of *onset* and progress of *neurological espisodes*.
2. Historical evidence of *coronary* or *limb atherosclerosis*

Examination

1. Full *clinical neurological examination.*
2. *Neck—*
     common carotid pulses
     external carotid pulses
         (facial, sup. temporal)
     bruit and *site of its maximum intensity but* remember it may
         occur in absence of atherosclerotic narrowing.
3. Evidence of *limb atherosclerosis* (absent pulses).

General investigations

As for limbs.

Special investigations

These may include ocular plethysmography, measurement of the direction of flow in the supraorbital branch of the ophthalmic artery, computerised axial tomography, dynamic gamma-imaging of the brain (brain scan), and ultrasound imaging of the carotid artery.

Carotid arteriography

Only on specific instructions.

Abdominal Aneurysm

Leaking abdominal aneurysms present with reasonable frequency to general surgical services.

1. *Suspect* the condition when pain has been sudden, is severe and unremitting, prominent in the back or legs and associated with a fall in BP. Beware the patient with 'left renal colic' who has pallor, tachycardia, and hypotension.

132

2. *Confirm* the suspicion by allowing the palpating hand to remain on the abdomen long enough to detect the *pulsating mass*; when in doubt, a supine AP and lateral views of the lumbar spine may show calcification in the aneurysm.

3. *Manage* the condition along the following routine lines. The mortality rate is high and the hope of bringing it down lies in being well prepared and able to follow a plan accurately.

4. If the patient is referred from elsewhere try to get the following information and action:

(a) Obtain as much of the past history as possible.

(b) Ask for the most urgent transfer.

5. While transport is awaited and or at the time of admission, as many of the following as possible should be done, but *must not delay* the patient's despatch from elsewhere:

(a) Insert a wide-bore IV cannula into the arm at or above the elbow.

(b) Blood group: phoning this ahead saves time.

(c) Draw blood for urea and electrolyte concentrations and phone results when available.

(d) Insert a self-retaining catheter into the bladder, and measure urine flow.

(e) Take a lateral X-ray of the abdomen.

(f) Send all X-rays and notes with the patient.

(g) Arrange for a doctor to accompany the patient.

6. Either at time of referral or if the patient is on your own service at once inform:

(a) Consultant surgeon on call.

(b) Theatre, and ask them to set up a urethral catheter and IV trolley if these have not been done.

(c) Casualty, particularly to tell them that the patient is to be taken straight from the ambulance to the anaesthetic room.

(d) Blood transfusion service to ask for 8 units of blood to be cross-matched.

(e) Duty anaesthetist.

7. When patient is in the anaesthetic room:

(a) Reassess: if diagnosis is thought to be incorrect transfer back to the ward; if diagnosis is thought to be established:

(b) Check efficiency of venous catheter, and establish a CVP line.

(c) Induce anaesthesia *without relaxation*.

(d) Explore abdomen, giving the patient relaxants only as the peritoneum is opened.

Arterial Embolus

The situation here has been transformed, so far as limb survival is concerned, by the introduction of Fogarty's embolectomy catheters. Limbs not actually gangrenous can frequently be saved by comparatively simple operations, under local anaesthesia if necessary.

Important practical points are:

1. Whenever a major embolus has possibly occurred, give *heparin* 5000–10000 u IV *before* detailed investigation: the major cause of failure in embolectomy is propagated thrombus.

2. While the patient's cardiac state is often poor, major limb or mesenteric gangrene is usually *lethal*.

3. Emboli can be removed from all limb arteries under *local or regional anaesthesia*.

4. In any patient with known mitral stenosis or atrial fibrillation who develops sudden, severe, abdominal pain—remember *mesenteric embolus*.

5. The commonest complication after embolus is another embolus, so that postoperative anticoagulation may be advisable.

Arterial Injuries

1. Arterial occlusion may be caused by blunt injury to the artery from *fracture*, rapid *deceleration*, or near-passage of a *missile*. It may be caused by penetrating injury that *severs* the artery, or that results in a *false aneurysm* which thromboses.

2. Whatever the precise cause, the limb or organ is in immediate jeopardy, with a time limit of *6 hours maximum* before irreversible damage occurs.

3. In any injured patient in whom arterial damage has been possible, *distal pulses* must be sought. If they are impalpable, an arterial occlusion must be assumed and must take *precedence* over all other injuries except those that are immediately life threatening.

Raynaud's Phenomenon

This term is used to describe a variety of conditions in which some or all of *pallor* or *blueness*, *pain*, and *coldness* occur in the fingers (and sometimes toes). These conditions can be divided into two subsets:

1. Recurrent episodes of a sequence of pallor—blueness—reactive hyperaemia affecting *all fingers of both hands* and associated with cold exposure, lasting minutes rather than hours, and with age of onset usually less than 20 years. This condition is common, often familial, most often affects females, is due to *cold-induced hyperreactivity* of the digital vessels, and has a uniformly benign prognosis. Occasionally the symptoms result from the use of *vibrating tools* or from *beta-blocking drugs*.

2. An episode of *pallor or blueness* and *severe pain* affecting only *one or a few fingers*, lasting days or weeks, with age of onset usually over 40 years. This is caused by *organic occlusion of digital arteries*, from any one of a wide variety of conditions the most common of which is *scleroderma*. The outlook is generally bad, with the risk of further episodes and digital tissue loss. Diagnostic tests should be performed for *scleroderma*, *blood disorders* including abnormal cryoproteins, and a source of *emboli* should be sought (notably subclavian plaque or aneurysm).

Complications of Arterial Surgery

There are many which may occur, but three of particular importance are:

1. *Sudden occlusion of a graft or prosthesis*. Since the collateral vasculature is usually unprepared, the viability of the distal tissues is often threatened and urgent treatment may be necessary.

2. *False aneurysm*, usually at the junction of a prosthesis with the artery and usually due to low grade infection. The manifestations may be *fever and local pain*; a palpable *aneurysm*; or *bleeding* from rupture of the aneurysm (including haematemesis and melaena from an aorto-duodenal fistula).

3. *Infection*. Apart from the local manifestations of false aneurysm, an infected graft may cause systemic symptoms not unlike subacute bacterial endocarditis.

17. VARICOSE VEINS

History

1. *Age of onset*
2. Relation of this to first *pregnancy*

3. *Number of pregnancies*

4. Past *superficial venous thrombosis*

5. Past *frank deep vein thrombosis*—white or blue swollen leg of pregnancy

6. Past *possible* deep vein thrombosis—? long period of recumbency

7. *Family history*—did *mother* and *father* have varicose veins?

Examination

1. Skin changes—
   eczema
   ulcer
   fat necrosis
2. Varicose vein distribution
   great saphenous
   small saphenous
   vulval or buttock
   combinations
3. Is there evidence of sapheno-femoral valvular incompetence: .
4. (a) Groin thrill or impulse on coughing
   (b) Varices controlled by high-thigh tourniquet
   (c) Low tension in varices with upright exercise and high-thigh tourniquet
4. Is there evidence of incompetent valves in perforating veins:
   (a) Subcutaneous fat necrosis
   (b) Palpable defects in deep fascia
   (c) Varices not controlled by mid-thigh tourniquet, and high tension in them with upright exercise and mid-thigh tourniquet
5. Are ankle pulses absent, suggesting concomitant arterial disease?
6. In an adolescent, are there skin haemangiomata and/or limb overgrowth indicating congenital arteriovenous fistulae?

Pre- and post-operative care

1. The varices must always be *marked* before operation—usually by the surgeon.
2. After operation there are only two postures permitted the patient:

(a) *In bed*, with the foot of the bed elevated.
(b) *Actively walking*.
The patient is *not* permitted to sit.

18. BREAST

Abscesses

These present certain difficulties in treatment. They are almost all staphylococcal. The patient will have received some sort of antibiotic therapy before being referred. They will generally have been present for from 1 to 4 weeks and are often *chronic thick-walled abscesses*.

There is a considerable tendency for further loculation of the abscess to occur with imperfect drainage. It is important to ensure that *all* loculi are broken down and all pus and dead tissue removed at the time of initial drainage.

Antibiotics are usually not helpful and should be in any case withheld till culture and antibiotic sensitivity are available.

Carcinoma

The premise to be followed is that *all* lumps in the breast which clinically are not definitely carcinomata are excised and examined macroscopically and microscopically. Where facilities are available, always warn the pathology department on the previous day that a frozen section may be requested. Sometimes, aspiration cytology will have given some indication of the diagnosis, but most surgeons will still regard it as essential to get histopathological confirmation. This can often be done using a needle biopsy technique under local anaesthesia (see p. 24). If the report is carcinoma, treatment can be proceeded with; if not, excision-biopsy must be performed.

History

Record:

1. Time for which lump has been noticed.
2. Nipple discharge or bleeding.
3. Pain and any relation to periods.

4. Lumps which have previously appeared and disappeared.
5. Children and circumstances of breast feeding.
6. Family history of Ca breast.
7. Detailed menstrual history for the last two years.

Examination

1. Examination of both breasts, axillae and neck. The *greatest diameter* of the breast lump in cm should be recorded. Its position within the breast, and the presence of *any* palpable axillary or supraclavicular lymph nodes should be recorded.
2. Palpable or impalpable liver.
3. Rectal examination—? palpable metastases.

Investigations

It is wholly inappropriate to try and 'cure' a patient with disease that is disseminated. Therefore considerable efforts should be made to establish if distant metastases are or are not present. A bone scintiscan may show 'hot spots'; these are then X-rayed. Liver function tests are probably as sensitive as liver scintiscan for hepatic metastases.

Preoperative management

1. Correction of anaemia as directed—opinions differ about acceptable levels of haemoglobin.
2. Crossmatch 2 units of blood.
3. NEVER use the ARM VEINS on the affected side for IV infusion or anaesthetic agents. Chronic swelling of the arm and hand is a dreadful complication.
4. Try to ensure that the patient is adequately counselled and comforted before this even more than most operations. A representative of a mastectomy society may be helpful and immediately after operation arrangements should be made for an external prosthesis.
5. Some treatment options involve radiotherapy. If so, it is best that the radiotherapist sees the patient before surgery.

Management

No one standard operation is at all widely accepted, but some form of mastectomy is likely to be carried out whenever the lesion is locally operable and no distant metastases are evident.

Postoperative care

Suction drains are now universally used. The tube is removed when the drainage has become minimal or after 10 days.

Rehabilitation

Aggressive physiotherapy for early arm movement is unnecessary.

19. GASTRO-DUODENAL SURGERY

Massive Upper GI Tract Bleeding

This is a common cause of hospital admission. Usually the patient tends to be managed first by a medical team, but surgeons are often involved. There is an increasing tendency to undertake joint management. The problem is twofold: (1) to control the circulatory insufficiency caused by blood volume reduction and often by coexistent cardio-pulmonary disorder in elderly patients; and (2) to identify the site of bleeding. In doing the first it is necessary to take into account the very real possibility that an elderly patient may have had a myocardial infarction, in which case transfusion necessary to correct anaemia must be cautious. In achieving the second, urgent endoscopy as soon as the circulation is stable is now generally recognised as better than urgent radiology. However, the latter may be necessary to confirm an endoscopic diagnosis or to follow on after a negative endoscopy.

So: Crossmatch adequate blood—6–8 units.

Do baseline investigations (p. 24).

Consider an ECG.

Arrange endoscopy in consultation.

Be prepared to follow on with arrangements for theatre or other treatment.

Perforated Peptic Ulcer

As soon as gastro-duodenal perforation is suspected the stomach is emptied and kept empty. Operative closure of the perforation and peritoneal toilet should be carried out as soon as the patient is fit for operation. Following perforation of a duodenal ulcer, the peritoneal contents are sterile, but only for the first few hours. The only exception to the rule of early operation is the patient whose general condition is so poor that operation offers a greater risk than conservative treatment with intravenous fluids, gastric suction and antibiotics. In practice, those who fall into the latter category are moribund.

History

Enquire for:

1. Convincing history of ulcer pain.
2. Recent exacerbation before perforation.
3. Previous radiological or surgical proof of an ulcer.
4. Previous or present haematemesis or melaena.
5. It is becoming increasingly important to enquire as to whether the patient has recently been receiving corticosteroids. If so, steroids must be administered as on p. 101 to cover operative period. Remember that perforation is commoner in those taking steroids.

Examination

1. A perforated peptic ulcer produces almost invariably right-sided or generalised abdominal tenderness with guarding amounting to rigidity. When the perforation is high on the lesser curvature or in the fundus of the stomach, the signs may be maximal on the left side. It is of the greatest importance to determine the *exact site of maximal tenderness and guarding*, for on occasions acute appendicitis is confused with a perforated ulcer. The two can in most cases be distinguished clinically by the fact that guarding in the former is maximal in the right lower abdomen and in the latter in the right upper abdomen.

2. Percussion to detect the presence or absence of normal liver dullness is of importance. The replacement of the normal liver dullness by a tympanitic note is diagnostic of a perforated hollow viscus.

3. It is important to perform a *rectal examination*, for in the presence of adynamic ileus, the detection of coincident bleeding may be possible only by inspection of the finger after withdrawal.

4. It is essential to assess the patient's *general condition*, both from the point of view of his present state and of long-standing cardiovascular or respiratory disease. On these findings must be based the decision whether to operate immediately, in an hour or two's time, or to practise non-operative treatment.

Investigations

1. In suspected perforated ulcer take a chest X-ray. It is by far the most sensitive way of detecting gas under the diaphragm.

2. Haematology screen if there is any evidence of anaemia or bleeding.

3. Cross-match two units of blood if it seems likely that a more major procedure than oversewing will be undertaken, or if there is evidence of coincident bleeding. *Gastrectomy* may be performed for gastric ulcer if the ulcer is very large, if it is a cancer, or if it is bleeding. *Vagotomy and drainage* or *highly selective vagotomy* may be done for duodenal ulcer if it is chronic, and this or gastrectomy if it is bleeding or stenosing.

Preoperative management

1. *Morphine* or *pethidine* should be given IM or preferably IV (see p. 19) as soon as the patient has been examined.

2. A *gastric tube* should be inserted and the stomach kept empty to reduce further leakage into the peritoneum.

3. An *intravenous infusion* should be set up before operation. Resuscitation with blood or plasma is rarely necessary, but may be so with late perforations.

4. Antibiotics are given. A cephalosporin (e.g. cephazolin 0.5 g immediately IV or IM and two further doses at 4 hourly intervals).

Postoperative management

This is identical to that for planned ulcer surgery below. When there is long delay between perforation and operation, the antibiotic may be continued for five days.

Postoperative complications

Subphrenic or pelvic abscess.
Wound infection.
Pulmonary collapse or infection.

Planned Ulcer Surgery

One of the important points is that peptic ulcers rarely kill. Therefore gastric surgery is not lightly undertaken, and every effort must be made to keep the complication and death rate to a minimum.

History

1. Total duration of ulcer symptoms.
2. Exact character of pain: situation, radiation, relation to meals, relief by alkalis, periodicity, etc.
3. Episodes of haematemesis, melaena, perforation.
4. Vomiting suggestive of duodenal or gastric stenosis.
5. The disability suffered by the patient with respect to work, etc. as a consequence of symptoms.
6. Details of past radiological diagnosis of peptic ulcer.
7. Details of previous medical or surgical treatment.
8. Dental state and efficiency.
9. Particular attention to matters important in the preoperative and postoperative management of the patient, i.e. respiratory, cardiovascular, genitourinary disorders.

Zollinger–Ellison syndrome (ZES) caused by a gastrin secreting tumour in pancreas or duodenum is a rare cause of peptic ulcer. Characteristically the ulcer disease is:
(a) Aggressive—i.e. has a short history.
(b) Leads to complications such as haemorrhage and perforation.
(c) Often multiple.
(d) Associated with other gastrointestinal symptoms such as diarrhoea.
The investigation of any such patient is vital because poorly planned surgery almost always results in a fatal outcome.

Examination

1. Local abdominal signs, particularly localised tenderness suggesting activity, as does the presence or absence of a gastric splash or visible gastric peristalsis.
2. Careful examination of cardiovascular and respiratory systems.
3. Examination of the mouth for dental sepsis.

Investigations

1. X-ray chest.
2. Haematology screen.
3. Biochemical screen, including electrolytes, blood urea, and albumin.
4. Have blood crossmatched.
5. Gastric secretory function tests are not used routinely but are indicated when Zollinger–Ellison syndrome is suspected. The features are:
(a) High resting secretion.
(b) Stimulated secretion is only slightly greater than resting.
6. Endoscopy should always have confirmed or reconfirmed the diagnosis before surgery is undertaken.
7. Plasma gastrin levels are done in:
(a) Suspected ZES.
(b) Recurrent ulcer, especially after gastrectomy.

Preoperative management

1. In order that the ulcer should be quiescent, anti-ulcer therapy using either antacids or H_2 receptor antagonists should be undertaken.
2. Correction of *dental sepsis* by conservative dentistry, extraction or fitting of dentures if required.
3. Deep breathing and leg exercises.
4. If there is gastric stasis from duodenal or gastric stenosis, daily evening *stomach washouts* with water or saline.
5. Insertion of *gastric tube* on the morning of operation.
6. An *intravenous drip* should be set up immediately before operation.
7. If the stomach is to be opened, preventative chemotherapy is used: e.g. cefazolin 0.5 g IM or IV with the premedication and two further similar doses at 4 hourly intervals.

Operative procedures

The standard procedures practised are:

1. Highly selective vagotomy
2. Selective or truncal vagotomy plus:
  (a) pyloroplasty
or (b) removal of the antrum and gastroduodenostomy
or (c) gastroenterostomy.
3. Partial or subtotal gastrectomy with gastro-duodenal anastomosis (Billroth I).
4. Subtotal gastrectomy with gastro-jejunal anastomosis (Polya type).

Postoperative management

1. The patient may require intravenous fluids and gastric suction for several days, especially after selective or truncal vagotomy. Gastric suction should range from hourly to four-hourly depending on the quantity aspirated. Intravenous fluid requirements are discussed in the appropriate section of this Guide (p. 86).

2. *Oral fluids* are started when the gastric aspirate is less than 200 ml per day, when bowel sounds are present and when the patient has passed flatus. Initially 30 ml per hour is given and the stomach aspirated four-hourly. The nasogastric tube should be removed as soon as the four-hourly aspirate is substantially below the oral intake. Since the stomach is readily aspirated by the gastric tube some surgeons start fluids by mouth after the first 24 hours. Some surgeons favour gastrostomy as a method of drainage. If a gastrostomy is used the tube should be left in until the stomach is firmly sealed to the abdominal wall—about 8 days.

Gastric Cancer

There is no satisfactory curative, or indeed palliative treatment for this condition other than surgery. From the point of cure, the results of surgery are poor. However, as with carcinoma of the large bowel, surgery offers excellent palliation of symptoms, and is undertaken whenever it is thought the patient's general condition permits gastrectomy and whenever it is *technically* feasible to resect the growth.

144

History

The important points are:

1. Previous dyspeptic symptoms.
2. Any comparatively recent change in the quality of the dyspepsia.
3. Vague symptoms, such as lack of appetite, lack of energy and more specifically, weight loss.

Examination

Abdomen. A search should be made for:

1. An upper abdominal *mass*.
2. Evidence of gastric obstruction in the form of *visible peristalsis* on a gastric *succussion splash*.
3. The presence or absence of a palpable *liver*.
4. The presence or absence of *ascites*.

Rectal examination (with particular reference to metastatic deposits in the recto-vesical or recto-vaginal pouch).

Examination of the neck for palpable supraclavicular lymph nodes.

Investigations

As for planned peptic ulcer surgery.

Preoperative management

In general this is as for a peptic ulcer and prophylactic antibiotics are indicated. Particular attention should be paid, however, to ensure that the patient receives during the preoperative period a *high protein*, *high calorie*, *high vitamin diet*, if necessary intravenously (p. 98).

Operative procedures

Total gastrectomy is the only satisfactory operation on theoretical grounds but is not commonly used.

1. For growths of the pylorus or body of the stomach an *extended subtotal gastrectomy* is performed, the extension consisting of the excision of the greater omentum, lesser omentum and lymph nodes along the vessels supplying the stomach, particularly the left gastric artery.

2. Palliative or curative resection of a carcinoma of the fundus of the stomach is technically feasible only by excising also the lower end of the oesophagus. In this instance, therefore, *oesophago-gastrectomy* by the thoraco-abdominal route must be performed.

Postoperative management

This is in all ways identical with that for peptic ulcer surgery and thoracic procedures.

20. BILIARY TRACT DISEASE

Cholelithiasis

Most patients will come in from the waiting list, almost always with a firm diagnosis of cholelithiasis, and will be for operation within the next two or three days. In documentation the important points are:

History

It is most important to obtain an accurate history of the exact nature of the attacks of acute pain, with particular regard to the *nature* of the pain, the *distribution* of the pain, associated symptoms such as vomiting, and the necessity or otherwise for pain relief. *Jaundice* must be enquired for, but it must be remembered that a high proportion of patients will state that they become 'yellow' during an attack. It is important to try to obtain objective evidence of jaundice, such as its observation by the general practitioner, or a quite definite association with *pale stools* and *dark urine*.

The occurrence of *fever* and *rigors* must also be enquired for, since rigors point to cholangitis and common-duct stones.

If there has been a previous *gall bladder operation*, the patient should be closely questioned about it and if possible full details obtained from the surgeon or hospital concerned: it does not follow that the gall bladder has been removed, even though the patient may think so.

Cholelithiasis is a common condition in countries with a high standard of living, and therefore the radiological demonstration of gall stones may mislead when the pain is due to some other lesion, e.g. hiatal hernia, peptic ulcer, cardiac ischaemia.

Examination

There are rarely abnormal physical signs referable to gall bladder disease and examination is therefore particularly directed at the fitness of the patient for operation.

Investigations

Operations on the biliary tract should be regarded as major procedures and a haematology and biochemical screen carried out as a routine. Chest X-rays and an ECG must also be done. In most instances the radiological diagnosis will have been made before the houseman sees the patient.

Postoperative management

1. Nil by mouth for 24 hours.
2. Removal of the drain after 1–2 days *unless there is drainage of bile*.
3. If a T-tube is in place, cholangiogram on the 8th day. Do *not* remove the tube till the film has been seen by the surgeon.

Postoperative complications

Bleeding. A moderate amount of blood may be lost through the drain postoperatively, but it is extremely rare for serious bleeding to occur.

Ileus. A mild adynamic ileus often occurs during the first 24 hours after operation. This is rarely of consequence, but if *vomiting* should persist, *abdominal distension occur* and bowel sounds not be detectable, *bile peritonitis* should be suspected. Bile peritonitis is insidious and is often not detected until jaundice from re-absorption becomes obvious.

Pulmonary collapse, followed sometimes by infection, is a not uncommon complication of cholecystectomy and probably accounts for the fever which frequently occurs in the first 48 hours.

Occult bile leakage. If bile should leak from the site of operation, it may fail to escape from the drain and accumulate first in the subhepatic pouch and then via the right paracolic gutter in the subphrenic space. The effect of this is to rotate the liver downwards to the left and so to obstruct the inferior vena cava. The clinical effects are thus often circulatory and the patient may show an insidious onset of circulatory inadequacy which may be confused with a myocardial infarction. Indeed, if myocardial ischaemic changes are already present they may become intensified as venous return is reduced, so making for a difficult ECG interpretation. As long as the possibility of bile accumulation is remembered, early drainage can be instituted.

Biliary Colic—Acute Cholecystitis

Common causes of emergency admission are patients with syndromes which range from acute biliary obstruction from a stone impacted in the cystic duct ('biliary colic'), through acute cholecystitis in which a bacterial element predominates, to acute pancreatitis of biliary origin. The last probably, but not conclusively, occurs because of a stone passing down the common bile duct. The gall bladder in such circumstances is nearly always non-functioning.

History

The important point is the dominance or otherwise of infection. This apart, the historical points worthy of record are similar to those for non-acute admissions.

Examination

Record:

1. The site of maximal *tenderness and guarding*.
2. The presence or absence of a *gall bladder mass*.
3. The presence or absence of *jaundice*.
4. *Fever*.
5. Presence or absence of *bowel sounds*.

Investigations

Within a few hours of admission attempts should be made to confirm the clinical diagnosis by:

1. Haematology screen, biochemical screen including liver function tests, serum amylase.

2. Blood culture if fever is marked or there is a history of rigors.

3. Plain X-ray of the gall bladder in an attempt to detect radio-opaque calculi—supine and erect films—and chest X-ray.

4. Ultrasound examination is the cheapest, most easily deployed method of detecting gall stones. It can also delineate an enlarged gall bladder and a dilated common duct. Its only flaw is that it is very 'operator dependent' and thus its reliability varies from hospital to hospital.

5. ^{99m}TcPG (or HIDA) biliary excretion scanning is, when facilities are available, the investigation of choice to establish that the gall bladder does not fill.

Management

The principal features of treatment in the initial phase are:

1. *Bed rest, parenteral fluids and pain relief.*

2. *Antibiotics* should *not* be given without consultation with a more senior member of the unit and are usually not necessary.

3. *Operation* is now quite frequently undertaken in the acute phase, usually at the next available operating session. It is certainly required if either systemic disturbance or local signs persist or advance. Acute pancreatitis (i.e. raised serum amylase—see p. 151) and co-existent biliary tract disease—evidence of jaundice or stones in the common bile duct from previous investigations—are also an indication for surgery.

Operative treatment is also indicated if there is co-existent cardiorespiratory disease. The risks of surgery are less than those of leaving a large inflammatory mass which impairs ventilation and decreases afterload.

4. If the acute attack subsides without surgery, *cholecystography* is arranged soon. If the diagnosis is confirmed radiologically, cholecystectomy is undertaken as soon as possible because there are risks of further attacks.

Obstructive Jaundice

The problem is often to differentiate between:

1. Biliary calculi.
2. Carcinoma—of ampulla, pancreas, or metastases in porta hepatis or liver.
3. Liver disease, especially that producing cholestasis (drugs, auto-immune hepatitis, rarely viral hepatitis).

When real difficulty exists in the differentiation on clinical grounds, liver function tests are, on the whole, of no further help. As with many other complex diagnostic problems a strictly logical sequence is useful.

Certain other investigations may help the differentiation of the conditions listed above and the decision to proceed to or withhold from laparotomy:

1. Faecal occult blood, if positive, suggests an ulcerating lesion of stomach or duodenum.
2. Gastroduodenal endoscopy may reveal a gastric or ampullary neoplasm, or suggest a pancreatic carcinoma and can be followed by retrograde cholepancreatography.

Thin needle *percutaneous transhepatic cholegraphy* (p. 50) carries with it only a very small risk of bile leakage and will delineate precisely the major bile ducts in most cases. Nevertheless, arrangements should be in hand for laparotomy if major bile duct obstruction is demonstrated.

Ultimately, if the jaundice is progressively deepening or fails to clear completely, *laparotomy* is usually undertaken.

Special precautions

Certain special precautions should attend laparotomy for jaundice, especially if the serum bilirubin is > 100 mmol/l:

1. All jaundiced patients should be given vitamin K analogue 20 mg daily from the time of admission. The prothrombin time must be measured the day before operation.
2. Antibiotic cover for operation using a cephalosporin or cotrimexalol should be routine to avert gram negative septicaemia. Whole-gut irrigation (p. 161) is used by some preoperatively to remove the organisms responsible for septicaemia.

3. Frusemide (40 mg IV) or mannitol (100 ml of 15% solution/ hour) should be administered preoperatively to maintain a brisk diuresis (greater than 60 ml/hour) and reduce the significant risk of renal failure.

21. ACUTE PANCREATITIS

The diagnosis of acute pancreatitis is very likely if a patient with acute upper abdominal pain has an amylase concentration in the blood in excess of 1000 iu/l. Exceptions are:

1. A few patients with perforated peptic ulcer or a strangulated loop of small bowel.
2. Afferent loop obstruction after Polya gastrectomy.

Thus, the differential diagnosis needs to be considered and the label of acute pancreatitis only applied after exclusion of these causes. Once acute pancreatitis has been diagnosed two things are important:

1. To establish a cause.
2. To grade the process for severity.

Cause

Gall stones and alcohol are the common ascribable causes. There may be a history which is suggestive. Gall stones can be detected by *ultrasound* or *plain film* and a non-functioning gall bladder by excretion scan (p. 52). Alcoholic pancreatitis may be supported by abnormal liver function tests and changes in the blood film suggestive of alcohol abuse (macrocytosis).

Examination and grading

Abdomen. Tenderness and guarding are usually diffuse. In general look for signs of shock and hypoxia. Measure serum concentration of amylase, calcium, glucose, arterial gas tensions, full blood count and urea and electrolyte concentrations, liver function profile. Do a chest and upright and supine abdominal X-rays (pulmonary involvement in the first and a 'sentinel' loop in the second).

A severe attack which may be fatal and certainly requires consideration of intensive care is defined in the first 48 hours by:

1. High blood glucose (greater than 11 mmol/l).
2. Raised white cell count (greater than 16×10^3 per μl).
3. Reduced arterial oxygen tension (less than 60 mmHg = 8kPa).
4. Acidosis.
5. Rising blood urea (above 16 mmol/l at 48 hours).
6. Falling haematocrit, and
7. Fluid requirement in 48 hours of more than 6 litres.
8. Progressive hypocalcaemia (less than 2 mmol/l).

Initial management

Set up a reliable intravenous line and in severe cases a central line to measure CVP. Administer Hartmann's solution to restore circulatory stability. Pass a nasogastric tube, institute nil by mouth and continuous aspiration. Do not administer 'specific' agents such as aprotinin (Trasylol) or glucagon unless instructed—the evidence supporting their value is thin.

Other investigations which may help establish a cause or assist in management:

Abdominal ultrasound for (1) gall stones, and (2) the development of serous accumulation in the lesser sac—a pseudocyst.

Biliary excretion scan shows non-filling gall bladder in acute pancreatitis of gall stone origin.

Continued management

Operation may be undertaken early in gall stone pancreatitis—consider having blood available. Assess ileus twice daily. Prolonged ileus is an indication to consider parenteral nutrition (p. 98). Otherwise, repeat investigations according to the following schedule:

Daily	*Twice weekly*
Urea and electrolytes	Liver function profile
Amylase	Ultrasound
Full blood count	
Gas tensions (until normal)	
Calcium (unless normal)	

22. INTESTINAL OBSTRUCTION

Small Bowel Obstruction

Opinions differ as to whether a trial of conservative treatment with intravenous fluid replacement and gastric suction should be undertaken. We believe that once the diagnosis is established, operative relief of the obstruction should be undertaken as soon as the patient's condition permits. It is not possible to distinguish definitely on clinical grounds between a simple mechanical obstruction and bowel strangulation. In the presence of strangulation delay contributes to the immediate higher mortality.

History

1. Duration, site and character of the *pain*.
2. The character of the *vomiting*—whether it be of small quantity and therefore reflex in type, or of large volume suggesting mechanical regurgitation.
3. When the patient's *bowels* moved last and when he last passed *flatus*.
4. The precise nature of any previous *abdominal operations* or *symptoms* suggestive of a *progressive bowel lesion*.
5. Enquire regarding the taking of *ganglion blocking or antidepressant drugs*.

Examination

Abdomen

1. Abdominal *distension* (often absent in early, *high* small bowel obstruction, or in *closed loop* obstruction).

2. Presence or absence of visible *peristalsis*.

3. Presence or absence of *tenderness and guarding*, suggesting strangulation.

4. Presence or absence of a *succussion splash*, particularly in the lower abdominal quadrants.

5. The character of the *bowel sounds*, and their relation to bouts of pain.

Examination for the presence of an incarcerated hernia, whether inguinal, femoral, umbilical or incisional.

Rectal and/or vaginal examination. Search for a pelvic mass of any description, and determine whether the rectum is full or empty.

Assessment of the patient's general condition to determine the amount of fluid replacement required. This is dealt with more fully under fluid and electrolyte replacement (p. 89).

Investigations

1. NEVER (as is sometimes recommended) order an enema. Your senior may rarely do so.

2. X-ray of the abdomen is important, even though the diagnosis is obvious. Take the X-rays before a sigmoidoscopic examination is considered. Air is insufflated at the latter investigation and may confuse the picture. One film should be taken with the patient *supine* and a second with the patient either *standing* or lying in a *lateral position*. It is important to include the *diaphragm* in the films. In general, the erect film is for the purpose of demonstrating *fluid levels* and confirming the clinical diagnosis; the supine film is to determine the *site* of the obstruction by means of the gas shadows in the bowel. Order a *PA chest* at the same time.

3. If time and circumstances permit, it is desirable to obtain haematologic and biochemical (electrolytes and blood urea) screens. However, as pointed out under the heading of fluid and electrolyte replacement (p. 90), with an obstruction of short duration these values may well be normal and give no guide as to the extent of the fluid and electrolyte loss which may have occurred.

154

Preoperative management

1. Administer a pain-relieving drug.
2. A naso-gastric tube is inserted, aspirated until the stomach is empty and placed on continuous drainage, but see p. 113.
3. An intravenous infusion is set up. In *acute* fluid loss there is no danger in rapid replacement, so at least half the estimated loss may be replaced rapidly, in the first one or two hours before operation (see p. 90).
4. In any case of intestinal obstruction do not rely on the naso-gastric tube to have effectively emptied the stomach. Be on hand at the time of induction of anaesthesia to carry out *cricoid compression* so as to avoid reflux and inhalation (see p. 114).

Postoperative management

This is almost entirely a question of fluid and electrolyte replacement and maintenance. Naso-gastric or gastrostomy drainage is continued until bowel sounds are present and/or the patient has passed flatus. Thereafter intake is rapidly built-up through clear fluids to mixed fluids to food.

Large Bowel Obstruction

With the exception of sigmoid volvulus, large bowel obstruction and its features tend to develop more slowly than in the case of the small bowel. The obstruction is essentially an acute-on-chronic type. Except where there is danger of rupture of the caecum there is therefore not the urgency with regard to operative treatment. Very occasionally conservative treatment is attempted, for if the bowel can be cleared and full bowel preparation carried out, planned surgery with a one-stage instead of a three-stage operation is feasible. However, there is currently a move to more aggressive resective surgery as an emergency or semi-emergency for the chief cause of large bowel obstruction—cancer.

History

1. It is most important to differentiate:
(a) *Acute volvulus* with sudden onset of severe abdominal pain, and often gross distension.

155

(b) *Diverticulitis* causing obstruction with a past history of similar attacks of pain in the left iliac fossa, fever, and possibly diarrhoea.

(c) *Carcinoma* which is the commonest cause of obstruction, with its attendant premonitory symptoms.

2. It is important to determine when the patient's *bowels* moved last and when he last passed *flatus*.

Examination

Abdomen

1. **Abdominal distension** of a large bowel (peripheral) type.

2. Evidence of a **localised abdominal** distension, i.e. is there a coil of sigmoid colon visible, suggesting a volvulus, or is the caecum visible, palpable or percussible?

3. The presence or absence of a *succussion splash*.

4. The presence or absence of *tenderness and guarding*— suggesting, according to the site, diverticulitis, sigmoid volvulus or danger of caecal rupture.

Rectal and/or vaginal examination. It is most important to attempt to detect the *obstructing mass*, whether carcinoma or diverticulitis.

Assessment of the patient's general condition. Vomiting is generally not prominent and while the patient may be ill, it is unusual for this to be due to gross fluid and electrolyte loss.

Investigations

1. Plain X-ray of the abdomen, as for a small bowel obstruction. The supine film is most important in determining the *site* of the obstruction from the gas shadows. *PA chest* at the same time.

2. If the diagnosis of actual large bowel obstruction is in doubt, or if the site and nature of the obstructing lesion is important to the proper selection of treatment, urgent barium enema should be mandatory. This may exclude patients with colonic 'pseudo-obstruction'—a dilated dysfunctioning colon, the result of multiple causes.

3. Sigmoidoscope the patient routinely but not until X-rays have been done. Gas inflation of the colon may distort the picture.

4. Haematology and biochemical (electrolytes and blood urea) screens should be undertaken. These are perhaps more important in the case of large bowel obstruction than small because pre-existing anaemia or uraemia are not uncommon.

Treatment

1. In the case of a *volvulus* of the sigmoid colon, decompression of the bowel and reduction of the volvulus can usually be achieved by the passage of a flatus tube through a sigmoidoscope.
If these measures fail or are not applicable, laparotomy must be performed.

2. (a) For a *carcinoma of the right side of the colon* an emergency right hemicolectomy is generally performed, therefore blood (4 units) must be ready.

   (b) For a *left-sided carcinoma* a right transverse colostomy or caecostomy will usually be done to decompress the bowel and permit planned resection some two weeks later. Alternatively, an immediate resection is carried out, with or without reconstruction.

   (c) For volvulus a *Paul-Mikulicz type of resection* may rarely be performed.

   (d) For an obstruction due to *diverticulitis* a decompressing colostomy is generally required and an associated abscess drained. Many surgeons now do an immediate resection of the sigmoid colon, with temporary end-colostomy and closure of the rectal stump.

Preoperative management

In acute large bowel obstruction this is as for small bowel obstruction except that prophylactic antibiotics are always *indicated. Suggested regimen:* Gentamicin 2 mg/kg and Metronidazole 500 mg are given IV 1–1½ hour preop. Consider two further doses of both drugs at 8 hourly intervals postoperatively. *Note* if Gentamicin is given postoperatively the dosage is 1 mg/kg.

Postoperative management

This generally presents less of a problem than with a small bowel

157

obstruction. Intravenous therapy may be expected to continue for only 24 to 48 hours. When the colostomy works, the patient may take oral fluids.

Further management, where definitive treatment has not already been carried out:

1. Resection of the obstructing lesion is carried out as soon as the laparotomy wound has healed. This is generally 2 to 3 weeks after the initial procedure. The pre- and postoperative management of this second procedure is as for planned surgery of the large bowel.

2. The final stage is closure of the colostomy, performed 2–3 weeks after (1).

23. LARGE BOWEL SURGERY

In common practice this is confined to a limited variety of resections. In former days, almost all of these would be preceded by a *defunctioning colostomy* in order to reduce the bacterial contents of the bowel to be resected. Nowadays, however, adequate bowel preparation may be carried out using principally mechanical cleansing of the bowel.

Preoperative Investigations

1. Usual haematology and biochemical screens. Preoperative blood transfusion given with the same indications as for gastric carcinoma.

2. Whenever possible a double contrast barium enema is done to exclude other disease in the colon.

3. As in all forms óf malignant disease, a *chest X-ray* should be performed. In the case of a lesion of the distal colon (unless it has previously been performed), a *sigmoidoscopy* to determine the precise *level* of the lesion, and for *biopsy*:

4. In the case of a lesion of the sigmoid colon or rectum, *an IVU should be performed*. This is to detect involvement of the ureters, and by means of a *post-micturition film*, to exclude significant urinary obstruction. The films also serve as a baseline by which to judge any postoperative urinary complications.

Stoma Management

The past few years have seen a minor revolution in the care of stomas—colostomy, ileostomy and occasionally ureterostomy. Not only have appliances and adhesives improved, but also nurses who specialise in these patients and their problems—stoma therapists—are increasing in number. When such a person is available she should be consulted *before* operation. She will share with the medical staff the burden of explanation to the patient (but remember it is difficult for anyone to comprehend a stoma until he or she has one) and map the site most suitable for the opening. Stoma therapists should work in concert with the surgical team not independently and their presence is not an excuse to subcontract.

Planned Procedures—Colon

Right hemicolectomy. For an obstructing lesion of the terminal ileum or right side of the colon as far as the hepatic flexure. Even in the presence of obstruction, this is carried out as a one-stage procedure.

Resection of the transverse colon. This may be either a primary planned resection, or resection following a decompressing caecostomy.

Left hemicolectomy or *sigmoid colectomy*. Again either a planned procedure, or following a right transverse colostomy or caecostomy.

Planned Procedures—Rectum

There are two standard procedures in use.

Anterior resection. This is a resection and end-to-end anastomosis with preservation of the lower rectum and sphincter, performed by the abdominal route. It is the procedure of choice in resection for sigmoid diverticulitis, and is used in selected cases of carcinoma. In general it is not employed unless the growth is more than 8 cm from the anus, in order that an adequate resection of normal bowel below the growth may be undertaken, and to retain normal bowel function. New stapling devices for making the anastomosis are pushing the limit down. The two chief dangers are:

1. Leakage at the suture line, which may not be evident till several days after operation and presents as a discharge of pus and faeces at the drain site, or as a pelvic abscess.

2. Obstruction at the anastomosis. On this account careful watch must be kept for abdominal distension for the first few days. A supine *abdominal X-ray* may be useful to distinguish small bowel distension (ileus) from large bowel (obstruction).

Abdomino-perineal resection. The simultaneous combined operation is undertaken, except where hip movement is so limited that adequate simultaneous exposure is impossible.

Preoperative Management

Mechanical bowel preparation

It is unwise and unsatisfactory to undertake definitive surgery on a loaded colon. Although it can sometimes be difficult to achieve, the prime objective of mechanical bowel preparation is to have an empty bowel.

If a decompressing colostomy has already been done, the patient's distal colon is washed out from the anus and through the colostomy until the return from both ends is clear; water may be used for this purpose. At the same time one of the regimens outlined below is used on the proximal bowel to reduce the problems of perioperative soiling of the abdominal wall.

In patients with intestinal continuity:

Technique A

On operation day minus 2:
Patient is admitted to hospital, eats a normal ward diet and that evening is given 2 bisacodyl tablets.

On operation day minus 1:
Has a normal breakfast but thereafter has a liquid diet. At 10 a.m. 350 ml of Magnesium Citrate Solution (U.S.N.F.) is sipped over an hour or so. That evening a phosphate enema is given.

Operation day:
Nil by mouth and at 6 a.m. the patient is given a high colonic lavage until the return is clear.

160

Technique B

Days Before	Diet	Aperients	Suppositories, Wash-outs
4	Ordinary	Mag. Sulph. 5 g each morning	2 bisacodyl suppositories in evening
3	Ordinary	Mag. Sulph. 5 g each morning	2 bisacodyl suppositories in evening
2	Light	Castor oil 45–60 ml at 6.0 a.m.	
1	Mainly fluid	Nil	Colonic washout or soap-and-water enema.
0 (Day of op)	Nil	Nil	Nil

Technique C (whole gut irrigation)

Operation day minus 1:

Pass nasogastric tube and place patient on commode. Infuse 10 l of Hartmann's solution down the tube at the rate of 3 l/h. This induces painless diarrhoea.

N.B. Do not use if obstruction is suspected or present and desist at once if pain is severe.

Whichever technique is used it should be routine to take a plain film of the abdomen on the afternoon of the day before operation. This is shown to the surgeon concerned so that he is satisfied with the absence of radiologically visible residual faeces.

Postoperative Management

With the exception of resections of the rectum, where special attention to the urinary tract and perineal wound is required, the postoperative management is much the same as for small bowel surgery.

Prophylactic antibiotics

Gentamicin 2 mg/kg and Metronidazole 500 mg are given IV 1–1½ hour preop. Consider two further doses of both drugs at 8 hourly intervals postoperatively. *Note* if Gentamicin is given postoperatively the dosage is 1 mg/kg.

24. GENITOURINARY SURGERY

Acute Urinary Retention in the Male

This is almost the most common urological emergency and its commonest cause is benign prostatic hypertrophy in elderly males. However, in any man suspected of having urinary retention it is always important to entertain the possibility of anuria which can be present even though catheterisation yields up to 300 ml of urine. It is imperative to record the volume of urine in the bladder and to follow output for six hours or so after the patient is catheterised so as to avoid confusing a low output with retention.

General investigation and initial management

History. Note the age of the patient. In a male under fifty be cautious in diagnosing prostatic obstruction and consider stricture. In any patient with urinary retention, ask about the nature of the stream, hesitancy, frequency of micturition by day and night and the ability of the patient completely to empty his bladder. Enquire for haematuria, symptoms suggestive of infection, previous urinary tract surgery, injury or instrumentation of the urethra. A detailed history of bowel function must be obtained. Ask whether the patient had been constipated recently, as constipation can be an important predisposing factor in the development of urinary retention in the elderly male with only minor prostatism. If any doubt exists as to the cause of retention, a careful neurological history must be taken with specific questions about sensory and motor function of upper and lower limbs. Enquire about previous back symptoms or injuries. It is also important to obtain information about the cardiorespiratory and central nervous systems for the assessment of the fitness and suitability of the patient for operation.

Examination. A thorough general examination is required and a number of special points should be emphasised:

1. A palpable bladder usually confirms the diagnosis of retention. A tender bladder suggests *acute* retention. A large non-tender bladder with dribbling from the penis (retention with overflow) suggests chronic retention, or may indicate a flaccid bladder.

2. The penis must be examined carefully to exclude a tight phimosis or a meatal stricture.

3. Rectal examination. To assess the size of the prostate a variety of reference standards have been used which range from grams to pieces of fruit. The absolute size of the gland is of importance only to the surgeon who is going to perform the operation. The consistency of the gland is the finding that requires the greatest attention. It is the feel of the gland that usually gives the first hint of carcinoma. Any hard nodule or a hard irregular prostate must be considered to be malignant until proven otherwise. It is important to remember that one is performing a rectal examination and not just feeling the prostate; examine the rectal mucosa, seminal vesicles and rectovesical pouch. If the prostate feels malignant, examine carefully for para-aortic and supraclavicular nodes, liver enlargement and bony tenderness, as the findings are important subsequently in the staging of the carcinoma.

Relief of retention

The first step in the treatment of most patients with retention is to obtain free bladder drainage, usually by urethral catheterisation. The following points are important:

1. Use a 16 or 18F Foley latex catheter with a 30 ml balloon. Smaller catheters tend to be too soft and to curl up in the urethra.

2. In an apprehensive patient use a small premedicating dose of intramuscular morphine (10 mg) and chlorpromazine (up to 25 mg) twenty minutes before the procedure.

3. Ensure as near absolute sterility as possible by:
   (a) using a 'no touch' technique
   (b) carefully retracting the prepuce and cleaning the glans with an aqueous antiseptic (e.g. hibitane). N.B. Replace the foreskin after catheterisation to avoid the risk of a paraphimosis.

4. Insert 10 ml of 1% lignocaine jelly into the urethra and hold it

there for 2–3 minutes by gentle finger pressure on the underside of the glans.

5. Test inflate the balloon of the catheter and make sure it forms a spherical shape.

6. Pass the catheter gently with a rotating motion.

7. When urine flows clamp the main channel and inflate the balloon to just less than the recommended volume. If the patient has pain the catheter is not fully in the bladder.

8. Connect the catheter to a closed drainage system. Though gradual decompression is often recommended to avoid haemorrhage from large vessels on the submucosa overlying the prostate, this is rarely practised.

Though perurethral catheterisation in prostatic obstruction is usually straightforward, occasionally a catheter will not pass. The problem can sometimes be overcome by the passage of sounds and the introduction of a catheter using a Foley introducer, but this approach can have disastrous consequences in inexperienced hands and should *not* be undertaken by a houseman. A false passage can be produced even by a soft catheter and injudicious attempts to pass instruments along the urethra will often only increase the problem.

In such circumstances it is preferable to resort to suprapubic catheterisation.

Suprapubic catheterisation

A number of suprapubic catheters are commercially available in kit form and are ideally suited for bladder drainage, although their bore is too small to cope with bleeding.

1. Do not attempt this procedure:
   (a) unless you are confident you know how to do it or have expert help
   (b) if there is a lower abdominal midline or paramedian incision to which bowel may be adherent
   (c) if the bladder is definitely impalpable.
2. Infiltrate with local anaesthetic (1% lignocaine).
3. Do not go more than 4 cm above the symphysis pubis.
4. Stay strictly in the midline.
5. If there is doubt about the size of the bladder a safe approach is to advance the 18 gauge needle in the midline to its full extent; at that

164

stage it is usually possible to feel the needle penetrate the bladder and this can be confirmed by withdrawing 1 or 2 ml of urine.

6. Insert as much tubing as possible into the bladder because as the viscus empties it falls away from the anterior abdominal wall and the end of the catheter may come out.

Special circumstances in acute retention

Constipation. Elderly frail men with mild prostatic hypertrophy may go into urinary retention if they become constipated. Unless they are in acute distress (and this is unusual) they should be initially treated by restoration of bowel function (for which a manual evacuation may be needed) and by mobilisation. Only if this fails should a catheter be passed.

Postoperative retention. There are three situations in the male:

1. Normal urethra but a painful perineal or lower abdominal procedure. Do not allow the bladder to become distended; if the patient cannot void after 16 hours pass a catheter, empty the bladder, relieve the pain and withdraw the catheter. Re-catheterisation is seldom necessary.

2. Same as above but mild or moderate prostatic hypertrophy. The catheter should be inserted as for the normal patient. However, it is best not to remove the catheter until the patient is able to stand, is reasonably active and has normal bowel function. If even then retention recurs then significant hypertrophy exists for which operation is required.

3. Damage to some component of the voiding mechanism, usually the motor nerves as a consequence of extensive pelvic dissection (e.g. abdomino-perineal excision of the rectum). Here retention should nearly always be anticipated and bladder drainage instituted. Recovery is slow and continued catheterisation may be required for 7–10 days.

Postoperative retention is much less common in the female. However, there are a number of elderly women with chronically distended bladders, the cause of which is often uncertain. They may *appear* to develop retention after operation. Usually such individuals should *not* be catheterised as prolonged bladder drainage may be required and serious infection ensue.

Stricture. The situation may be apparent from the history (e.g. past trauma; sexually transmitted disease; the slow onset of difficulty in a young man) or may be diagnosed at catheterisation by failure of the catheter to progress as far as the prostate. At all costs avoid further damage. Unless you have been trained do not yourself undertake dilatation. Decompress suprapubically and seek help.

Subsequent management of retention

Benign prostatic hypertrophy. In nearly all instances some form of prostatectomy should be undertaken as soon as possible. There is no need for 'emergency' prostatectomy; schedule the patient for the earliest operation list and thus avoid the complications of hospital, bed rest and prolonged catheterisation—respiratory infections, venous thrombo-embolism and urinary tract infection.

The obstruction caused by the prostate can be overcome by either a transurethral or an open operation. There has been a very marked swing towards transurethral surgery. Open operations tend now to be performed only if the gland is very large or if there are multiple bladder stones in association with diverticula. Transurethral resection of the prostate is usually carried out under spinal or epidural anaesthesia. This has the advantage of causing minimal respiratory problems and it is often possible to detect complications at an earlier stage than would be the case if a general anaesthetic had been used.

Investigation and preparation for operation

The following investigations are the minimum which should be undertaken:

1. To assess renal function—serum creatinine, urea and electrolyte concentrations.
2. Urine culture at the time of catheterisation to ensure that there is no infection.
3. Haemoglobin or haematocrit to ensure that the patient is not anaemic, particularly if there is a significant degree of uraemia.
4. Blood group and match two units, though in some centres where blood is readily available grouping alone may be acceptable.
5. Chest X-ray.
6. Intravenous urogram. The value of this investigation is debat-

166

able. It is unlikely to alter the need for or type of operation in benign prostatic hypertrophy and its main benefit will be to detect coexistent abnormalities. If there is a history of haematuria, recurrent infections or suspicion of a carcinoma of the prostate, then IV urography should be performed as it will help in diagnosis or staging.

7. Serum acid phosphatase concentration should be estimated if a carcinoma may be present. The enzyme is not of *diagnostic* value. Its major role is as a tumour marker to monitor the progress of treatment of carcinoma of the prostate.

8. Prostatic biopsy. If the prostate feels malignant either aspiration or needle biopsy should be undertaken (p. 24). Either a transperineal or transrectal approach can be used, but if large needles are employed transrectally an antibiotic which is effective against gram negative organisms should be given for 12 hours.

9. To this list of investigations may be added an electrocardiogram. However, the requirement for this usually depends on the patient's history and the wishes of the anaesthetist.

10. The other important aspect of preparation is to explain to the patient the nature of the operation, by which route it will be performed and also that after the operation there will be significant amounts of blood in the urine for up to 2 weeks. It is also essential to allay fears regarding potency following prostatectomy, but to explain that retrograde ejaculation is an almost invariable sequel.

Carcinoma of the Prostate

Even if the diagnosis of carcinoma of the prostate is made preoperatively it is probably still better to resect a passage than to treat with oestrogens for 10 to 14 days in the hope that this will cause sufficient shrinkage of the gland to overcome obstruction. A reasonable plan is to undertake, where medically possible, transurethral resection of the prostate in all men who present with retention due to a carcinoma. If the serum acid phosphatase is normal and a bone scan negative, surgery should be followed after 6 weeks by radiotherapy to the prostatic fossa and draining lymph nodes. The reason for waiting 6 weeks is to allow the prostatic fossa time to heal, as earlier irradiation will often lead to distressing frequency and urgency. It is also necessary to exclude infection before starting radiotherapy.

If the acid phosphatase is elevated or the bone scan is positive, or there is evidence detected by other means of spread beyond the prostate, radiotherapy should be abandoned in favour either of oestrogens, which should be given in a dose of 1 mg stilboestrol 3 times a day, or orchidectomy which will have substantially the same effect. There seems to be no place for a larger dose of oestrogens as maintenance therapy for this condition. A departure from this regimen should be considered only in the presence of severe ureteric obstruction with uraemia. In these circumstances it has been thought that high doses of oestrogen in the form of the synthetic agent fosfestrol (Honvan), 1 g per day for a week, may *produce rapid shrinkage of the tumour and restoration of renal function*. Unfortunately this treatment has a high risk of venous thrombosis and heparin prophylaxis should be instituted (p. 109) at the same time as fosfestrol therapy. Although androgen suppression has been the mainstay of treatment, it is possible that it may be supplemented in the future by chemotherapy or used more frequently in conjunction with chemotherapy.

Management after transurethral and open prostatectomy

The bladder is kept free of blood by means of catheter drainage, using a 24 or 26F Foley catheter. Some surgeons prefer to use a continuous irrigation system, relying on the free flow to prevent clotting. An irrigating system, however, is of little use once clots have occurred and in these circumstances it is better to use a non-irrigating system. An alternative method for managing patients postoperatively is to use a fluid load, together with diuretics, to ensure a good urine output. This has the slight disadvantage that it may result in disturbances in fluid and electrolyte balance if not carefully managed, particularly in elderly patients.

Management of complications after prostatectomy

Hypotension. Probably the most common problem confronting a house surgeon following prostatectomy is hypotension. The major causes are blood loss and clot retention, bacteraemia and (less commonly) myocardial infarction. The first step is personally to check the recordings of temperature, blood pressure, pulse rate and to assess whether there is peripheral vasoconstriction. Then examine the catheter to see if it is draining adequately and the nature of the fluid coming out and examine the abdomen to see if the bladder is distended.

Blood loss. The fact that blood loss is the cause of hypotension is usually easily established. There will be a history of heavily blood stained urine postoperatively with difficulty in maintaining drainage and both will be apparent when the catheter bag is examined. There will often be clot retention (see below). In these circumstances it is necessary to replace blood, to ensure that there is free drainage from the bladder and to remove clots by bladder washout. If the closed drainage system has to be broken several times to wash out the bladder, antibiotics should be given systemically.

Clot retention. In spite of the measures outlined above, bleeding can still be sufficiently severe to cause clots to form and hence lead to retention. Do not be misled by clear through-and-through drainage because often the clot prevents the irrigating fluid from reaching the bladder. Pain should be relieved by small doses of opiate (see p. 20). The clots can usually be cleared by a vigorous bladder washout using either normal saline or citrate solution. Many simple manoeuvres such as letting down the balloon of the Foley catheter, or pushing the catheter further into the bladder, may be tried to improve drainage. In general, it is preferable not to remove the catheter unless an experienced person is available or has advised this because it may be very difficult to re-insert a catheter, particularly after transurethral resection of the prostate. If the bleeding is so severe that adequate drainage cannot be maintained and clot formation persists, the patient will have to be prepared for return to theatre and either washouts under anaesthesia or direct attempts to control the bleeding will then be made. Sometimes bleeding in the immediate postoperative period can be controlled by over-inflating the Foley balloon with 40–50 ml of water and placing the catheter under traction—in some centres this is routine.

Bacteraemia. It is important always to be on the alert for this complication. The urinary tract is without doubt the most common source of bacteraemias. Patients should *not* undergo endoscopic or any other surgery on the prostate in the presence of an untreated infection. The patient's temperature will be raised, he will have a tachycardia and possibly rigors; there will be a fall in blood pressure and peripheral cyanosis. When called to see such a patient it is important to assess his general condition, to ensure that he has an adequate fluid input, to take blood for blood culture and to give the 'best guess' antibiotic parenterally. Check that a urinary tract infection has not been overlooked before surgery. Organisms present in a preoperative culture will point to the correct diagnosis and also help in the selection of antibiotics to treat this condition.

For patients in severe shock it may be necessary to insert a central venous pressure catheter and to transfer them to an intensive care unit so that more intensive monitoring of cardiorespiratory function can be done. The condition requires rapid, aggressive treatment as it is potentially lethal (see p. 124).

Complications of transurethral resection

Blood loss is more easily underestimated in endoscopic than in open prostatectomy because of the large volumes of irrigating fluid involved. Care must be taken to examine the irrigating fluid during operation and because one is often dealing with frail, elderly men, blood replacement should be instituted before there are gross changes in pulse rate and blood pressure.

Fluid overload. Because of the nature of irrigating systems used during transurethral resection, large amounts of the irrigating fluid can be forced into the prostatic vessels and thus the systemic circulation. This can be minimised, but not totally prevented by keeping the fluid reservoir no more than 70 cm above the operating table. Most units now use a glycine solution which is isotonic. However, in some centres water is still used. In the case of glycine solution, a dilutional hyponatraemia occurs and if water is used, this is aggravated by red cell lysis. Often the first indication that excessive fluid absorption is occurring is that the conscious patient under regional anaesthesia becomes agitated, restless and confused. The operation should be stopped, blood sent for serum sodium concentration and osmolality estimations and 2% saline given intravenously. A large dose of a diuretic such as frusemide should be given intravenously as this will produce a diuresis with excretion of water in excess of electrolytes.

Bladder rupture or capsular perforation. Both these conditions are usually detected during operation. The usual features are that the

170

patient begins to complain of pain and the irrigating fluid does not seem to be returning properly. In these circumstances it may be necessary to make a suprapubic incision to drain the extravasated fluid and if necessary, repair the damage to the bladder.

Renal Calculi and Renal Colic

Stones in the urinary tract are also a common cause of acute surgical admission. Usually the patient has a stone arrested somewhere between the pelvi-ureteric junction and the bladder.

The diagnosis of a ureteric calculus as a cause of severe abdominal pain is usually clear from the history, although at times this disorder may be confused with biliary colic, intestinal obstruction, appendicitis, leaking aortic aneurysm, hysteria, or a twisted ovarian cyst. There is a small group of patients who simulate renal colic in order to obtain narcotics (p. 57). It is important to confirm the diagnosis as soon as possible, both in order positively to exclude other dangerous lesions and also to establish the effects the stone is producing on the kidney. If investigation is delayed the stone may pass so that when X-rays are taken nothing is found and the diagnosis remains in doubt.

Investigations

Microscopical examination of the urine. This should be performed on the first specimen of urine obtained. Almost invariably there will be red cells in the urine in the presence of renal colic. Although red cells *can* be absent, this finding casts doubt on the diagnosis.

Urine culture. It is important to exclude concurrent infection as the combination of complete or partial obstruction and infection can have rapid and disastrous effects on the kidneys.

Haematological and biochemical studies, particularly serum creatinine and calcium concentrations, should be obtained on admission.

An intravenous urogram should be performed as soon as possible. This allows one to establish the diagnosis, to determine the size of the stone and also to tell the patient the likely course of management. In general, the size of the stone determines the management of the patient, assuming one is not dealing with specialised cases such as a solitary kidney or a stone in the presence of infection. When there is diagnostic doubt or urgency it is proper to undertake a urogram without the usual preparation which aims to remove overlying gas. The objective is less a precise anatomical diagnosis than to seek supportive evidence for the presence of ureteric obstruction. A 5, 10 and 30 minute film suffices and compression of the abdomen is not necessary. Thus, the examination can be performed with the emergency room X-ray facilities. Always make the point on the request form that the purpose of the investigation is to get a diagnosis when there is doubt. The three important signs on the affected side are:

1. Delayed excretion
2. A 'nephrographic' effect—contrast medium outlining the renal substance
3. An 'open' ureter down to the site of the obstruction, rather than the usual spindle.

Management of renal colic

Conservative.
1. Pain relief. Pethidine provides adequate pain relief, but it is important to make sure that enough is given. Too often, small incremental doses are used which do not adequately overcome the pain. In fit young men 100 mg IM or an initial 50–70 mg IV should be the minimum dose.
2. Ensure that there is adequate fluid intake. This may not always be easy as there is frequently a degree of ileus associated with renal colic; it may then be necessary to give fluids intravenously.
3. Physical activity. Where possible the patient should be encouraged to remain ambulant.

Operative. In most instances the stone will pass spontaneously and as a working guide one can assume that 95% of stones of less than 5 mm in diameter will pass spontaneously, whereas only about 5% of stones greater than 10 mm in diameter will do so. The other major indications for surgery—removing the stone either endoscopically (preferred) or at open operation—apart from size are:

172

1. A co-existent urinary tract infection.
2. A solitary kidney with impaired renal function.
3. Persistent severe pain with no radiological evidence of movement of the stone.
4. No symptoms, but where the stone has failed to progress over a period of no more than 6–8 weeks.

All patients who are to undergo surgery for stone should have a plain X-ray film of the whole renal tract on the way to operation.

Late management

Intravenous urogram. If a patient is being treated non-operatively it may be necessary to repeat the intravenous urogram, but in most cases a plain X-ray film is sufficient to show the progress or otherwise of opaque stones. If an operation has been performed it is important to ensure that there is free drainage and that the ureter has healed adequately following operation. Ultrasound imaging may prove satisfactory for follow-up because in most cases one is seeking the resolution of the pelvicaliceal dilatation caused by obstruction.

Urinary tract infection. Infection has to be excluded, but this largely applies to the follow-up of patients who have had staghorn calculi removed. In most other circumstances, unless there is some clinical indication, there should be no need to undertake routine urine cultures.

Biochemical investigation. The important objective is to find out if the patient has hyperparathyroidism. There are many ways of going about this but repeated serum calcium concentrations are the first line of investigation. At least three should be done over 2–3 weeks.

Treatment. After the first stone episode the patient should be advised to try to maintain a urine output of 1–1.5 litres per 24 hours. It is important to stress to the patient that their fluid intake is relatively irrelevant and that the important factor is their urine output. They should also be advised regarding diet, particularly those who have had calcium/oxalate stones. It is valuable to have available to a diet sheet which lists the foods which are rich in calcium and oxalate.

Recurrent stones. The management of patients with recurrent stones may be helped by more extensive metabolic studies under controlled conditions and, depending on the findings, stone recurrences may be prevented by treatment with such agents as thiazides, cellulose phosphate or allopurinol.

Major Surgery on the Urinary Tract

Apart from prostatectomy, already considered, and major operations on the kidney, the management of which corresponds to other abdominal procedures, the other major surgical assault is total cystectomy for bladder cancer. This operation may be difficult and bloody and involves, because of the ileal conduit, a change in life style. The following apply:

1. Make the patient aware of the problems of the ileal conduit and if there is a stoma service, enlist their help.
2. Warn the male patient of the inevitability of impotence.
3. Order 6 units of blood.
4. Discuss preventative chemotherapy with the surgeon (p. 66).
5. Arrange bowel preparation (p. 160).

25. TRANSTHORACIC SURGERY

In a general surgical unit the most common conditions for which a thoracic approach is used are hiatal hernia, carcinoma or stricture of the lower end of the oesophagus, and carcinoma of the cardiac end of the stomach. In the first of these conditions a purely thoracic approach will be employed, in the others an abdomino-thoracic.

Preoperative management

1. Great attention must be paid to *preoperative breathing exercises* so the patient may establish a routine which is carried on after operation. An attempt should also be made to correct any specific abnormality of ventilatory function (see pages 4 and 103).
2. Stop the patient smoking.
3. Treat any existing lung infection.
4. Assess respiratory function by VC, FEV_1, and baseline arterial blood gases.

Postoperative management

Underwater drain. The purpose of this is to ensure that a negative intrapleural pressure exists and therefore full lung expansion will result, while permitting the drainage of blood or exudate. The fluid level in the drain will normally fluctuate with respiration; if it does not, either:

1. The lung has fully re-expanded and is blocking the end of the draining tube, in which case no action is required, or
2. The drain itself is blocked with blood clot and will require clearing by milking its contents, by suction, or rarely by carefully controlled irrigation. A chest X-ray will usually resolve the problem.

Rules for removal of the chest drain vary from unit to unit.

General guidelines: full expansion demonstrated radiologically for 24 h; output of serum less than 50 ml/24 h; no concurrent need for drainage, e.g. an anastomosis.

The lungs should be fully expanded within a few hours of operation and remain so. Therefore a *chest X-ray* must be taken and inspected on the *evening of the operation*, on the *two successive days* and at less frequent intervals until the patient is fully convalescent. If at any time there are clinical and radiological signs of *pulmonary collapse*, urgent measures must be taken. The first is the active *personal* encouragement of the patient to cough up retained sputum. If this produces improvement conservative measures are persisted with and may include 'tracheal suction'. If there is, however, no improvement, immediate *bronchoscopy* may be necessary and advice should be sought.

26. THYROID AND PARATHYROID SURGERY

Thyroid

History

1. **Duration** of the goitre and *recent change in its size,* as well as *recent change in voice, difficulty with swallowing, cough, shortness of breath,* etc.

2. Cardinal symptoms of **hyperthyroidism** should be enquired for.

3. What **drugs** have been taken? For how long?

4. The *locality* in which the patient was born and spent his early life should be recorded, together with the presence or absence of goitre among other members of the *family*.

Examination

1. The *size* of the goitre.

2. Its *consistence*, and whether it is *diffuse or nodular*.

3. Is there an *intrathoracic extension*? Make the patient cough.

4. Is there *tracheal compression*, as judged by wheezing on hyperextension or other movement of the neck?

5. Is there *voice change* suggestive of recurrent laryngeal nerve involvement?

6. Is there a *Horner's syndrome* suggestive of cervical sympathetic involvement?

7. Is there clinical evidence of *hyperthyroidism*?

Investigations

1. Haematology screen.

2. **PA chest** and *views of thoracic inlet* for tracheal compression.

3. **Laryngoscopy** by arrangement with the ENT Department.

(a) A cord palsy *may* signify carcinoma.

(b) As a record to compare with postoperative appearance.

4. **Ultrasound** to delineate cysts.

5. **Hyperthyroidism.** In most patients the diagnosis will have been established but if investigations are required:

(a) Sleeping pulse rate.

(b) Thyroid function tests (remember to enquire about recent iodine intake by mouth, exposure to iodine-containing radiocontrast media, oestrogens or contraceptive pill).

6. **Scanning**. A thyroid gamma scan is not now generally regarded as vital, but from time to time gives useful information on two counts:

(a) Anatomy.

(b) The presence or absence of uptake in the nodule or nodules. If a 'cold' nodule is revealed by gamma scanning, a cyst may be distinguished from a solid tumour (? neoplasm) by ultrasound scanning.

Preoperative preparation

In most patients no special preparation will be required. In hyperthyroid patients the preparation will generally have been carbimazole 30–60 mg daily plus thyroxin 0.3 mg daily until the patient is euthyroid. Preoperative preparation may also include 10 drops of Lugol's iodine solution t.d.s. for 10 to 14 days to make the gland less vascular and a beta-blocking drug such as propranolol. Some units rely entirely on propranolol given in doses of up to 120 mg/day controlled by the resting pulse which should fall to below 70 per minute.

When the patient has a solitary nodule, frozen section should be arranged.

Postoperative management

This is in most cases uncomplicated. There are certain complications, however, which require emergency treatment.

1. **Haemorrhage** into the pretracheal space with asphyxia. The emergency treatment consists of the immediate removal, in the patient's bed, of skin and deep sutures to permit separation of the strap muscles and evacuation of clot.

2. Bilateral **recurrent laryngeal nerve damage** is very rare but may produce sufficient restriction of airway to necessitate emergency tracheostomy.

3. **Hypoparathyroidism.** This may occasionally occur as a complication particulary of total thyroidectomy for carcinoma and laryngo-pharyngectomy. After such a procedure is undertaken, a biochemical screen which includes serum calcium concentration should be done at first daily, and later less frequently. A watch should be kept at least daily for signs of impending tetany. Ask the patient if he/she has a feeling of tingling around the mouth. If so, tap the facial nerve gently with the finger tip. A twitch in the facial muscles suggests hypocalcaemia.

   (a) If frank symptoms and signs of hypoparathyroidism develop rapidly, give a slow intravenous injection of 10 ml of 10% calcium gluconate repeatedly if necessary.

   (b) For long-term therapy, give 4 to 20 g calcium by mouth daily as effervescent tablets or calcium tartrate powder (not tablets as they are not absorbed). Calciferol 100 000 units daily or dihydrotachysterol (A.T. 10) 0.75–2.5 mg daily (3–10 ml or 6–20 capsules).

4. In the unlikely event of a thyroid crisis or storm occurring: cold sponging or ice bath, IV saline, oxygen, morphine 15 mg and summon help. The most important and most specific treatment is propranolol 0.5–1 mg IV.

Parathyroid

The pre- and postoperative management for parathyroid surgery is much the same as that for thyroid surgery. Frozen section during operation is almost always needed. Postoperative hypocalcaemia is probable.

27. SKIN GRAFTS

Skin grafts are used for one of two reasons:

1. Trauma, including burns.
2. Replacement of skin following removal of a neoplasm.

Major non-urgent plastic surgery or cosmetic surgery is referred to a specialist plastic surgical unit.

The following are commonly used:

Split skin grafts. Taken with a Humby or Braithwaite knife or electric dermatome. Donor area is generally thigh, which *must be shaved*. Split skin grafts may be harvested but not applied immediately. They are kept in the Blood Bank refrigerator (not frozen) wrapped in saline-moistened gauze in a wide-mouthed sterile container. They can be used, as temporary or permanent cover, for up to 14 days and do not require sutures.

Free full thickness graft. This is generally taken from behind the ear and is used chiefly for the face.

Pedicle grafts. These are sometimes used in finger or hand injuries.

The dressing of a skin graft should always be left in the first instance to the surgeon in charge of the patient.

28. TRAUMA

Head Injuries

History

It is important to obtain from the ambulance driver, relatives, or from the Casualty Officer, a history of *changes* in the state of consciousness from the time of injury until the patient is seen.

Examination

Free airway. First and all the time.

Local injury. Never forget that a *scalp laceration* may cover a *compound skull fracture*. Suture of a scalp laceration must be accompanied by examination of the depths of the wound and of the underlying bone if it is exposed. Examine the scalp closely for local *bruising*—it may overlie fracture and may be of importance in the decision as to which side to place initial burr holes.

Palpate the skull for a depressed fracture.

Examine the external auditory meatus, nares and nasopharynx for *bleeding or CSF*.

General examination

It is important to establish a 'neurological baseline' against which any subsequent observations are considered. It is of almost equal importance to establish other baseline observations, so that changes in condition which reflect other injuries may be correctly interpreted.

1. Level of consciousness.
2. State of pupils.
3. Active movement of limbs and reflexes.
4. Blood pressure, heart rate, respiratory rate.
5. Associated injuries. Never forget that the head injury may not be the only significant one, and that the unconscious and even the conscious patient may not be able to describe the remainder. Thus look for
   (a) Fractured *facial bones*

179

(b) Fracture or dislocation of *cervical*, *thoracic*, or *lumbar spine*
(c) Fracture of the *clavicle*
(d) *Upper limb* fractures
(e) *Rib* or *sternal* fractures
(f) *Examine the abdomen*—local guarding is an important sign in the unconscious patient—but recourse to peritoneal lavage may be required (p. 185).
(g) Test the stability of the *pelvis*
(h) *Lower limb* fractures.

Investigations

Skull X-ray pictures (see section on *X-rays*). If the patient is admitted because of the risk that complications may develop rapidly, it seems reasonable to discover the skull fracture so that if intracranal bleeding should occur the probable side is identified. X-rays should be obtained on the way to the ward, *unless* the patient is so uncooperative as to make this technically impossible, or unless the patient is so *ill* that it is inadvisable for him to wait in the X-ray Department.

CT scan. This is a specialised investigation (see p. 55) but is now the definitive method of assessment in closed injury. Indications: focal signs, deteriorating consciousness.

Management

Free airway. In the unconscious patient this nowadays should mean an endotracheal tube, with or without assisted ventilation.

Observation.
1. *Level of consciousness* is the most important observation. Progressive loss of consciousness is perhaps the most reliable sign of cerebral compression.
2. *Pupils*. Pupillary changes when the patient is fully conscious *may* be of no significance. On the other hand, changes associated with change in the depth of consciousness may be of the greatest significance.
3. Regular *pulse and blood pressure* recordings should be routine. A slowing heart rate and rising BP strongly suggests cerebral com-

pression. Conversely, an accelerating heart rate and falling BP may indicate hidden blood loss or some other catastrophe.

The important observational matters have been integrated by Glasgow neurosurgeons into a coma scale which consists of three major components:

1. Eyes open: spontaneously; to speech; to pain; not at all.
2. Best verbal response: orientated; confused; inappropriate; incomprehensible; none.
3. Best motor response: obeys command; localises pain; flexion response to pain; extension response to pain.

Care of the unconscious patient. Do not forget the details of:

1. Free airway.
2. The patient should be nursed in an intensive care or high dependency unit, or be constantly attended by a special nurse. It is not sufficient to have state of consciousness, pupils, pulse and BP recorded or a coma scale filled in: clear instructions must be given as to the basis on which changes should be reported to you.
3. If the patient remains unconscious for more than a few hours, *bladder catheterisation and intravenous fluids* will be necessary. It is usual to restrict fluids to 1–1.5 l a day in head injury patients.
4. To protect the *skin* and encourage drainage of *bronchial secretions* the patient must be turned at least 4 hourly.

Sedation. In the disturbed patient this must be given with care, lest it disguise genuine changes in the level of consciousness. Each unit has its own preferences, but chlorpromazine or diazepam in small IV or IM doses have now largely replaced the traditional paraldehyde. Sometimes severe headache (e.g. from subarachnoid haemorrhage) is the basis of the disturbed state, and a non-narcotic analgesic may be more effective e.g. pentazocine 30 mg IM.

N.B. *Restlessness is not uncommonly due to a full bladder.*

Antibiotics. When there is certainty or suspicion of a *compound skull fracture*, these should be routinely given in the form of penicillin and Gentamicin if the patient is unconscious, or penicillin and sulphonamides if he can swallow.

Steroids. Dexamethasone (up to 40 mg daily), as a method of limiting post-traumatic cerebral oedema, has almost become routine. The evidence to support its use is not very good but provided its major side effects—failure of wound healing and gastrointestinal bleeding—are remembered, it can be used with safety.

Chest Injuries

Their importance lies not so much in the anatomical nature of the lesions, as in their effect on present and future respiratory function.

Examination

1. **Rib fractures** are detected by systematic palpation for local pain or crepitus.

2. It is most important to look for *paradoxical movement* of portions of the rib cage: *flail chest*.

3. **Tension pneumothorax,** or increasing pneumothorax, must be watched for (see p. 119). Subcutaneous emphysema *per se* is of no greater importance.

4. The presence of, or an increasing degree of, *haemothorax* must be assessed and drainage instituted.

Investigations

P.A. or A.P. portable chest X-ray is most important. It is unnecessary to ask for special views to detect rib or sternal fractures, as these are detectable clinically, and their significance lies only in the lung damage produced or the disorganisation of respiratory function.

Supine films may not show even substantial amounts of intrapleural blood and are condemned.

Watch particularly for the broadening of the mediastinum which may be due to a tear of the aorta.

In all except the most trivial injuries baseline (and usually repeated) arterial blood gas studies should be done.

Treatment

1. **Deep breathing** and **coughing** up of retained sputum.

182

2. **Antibiotics** at the first suspicion of pulmonary or pleural infection.

3. **Analgesics.** These should be selected and given with care in order that the cough reflexes should not be abolished. 2–5 mg of morphine may be given IV at 2 to 3 hourly intervals, or morphine may be given by continuous IV infusion (see p. 20).

4. **Rib fracture:** analgesics—chest strapping is of little value.

5. **Flail chest** with underventilation: endotracheal intubation and mechanical ventilation for 10–14 days.

6. **Tension pneumothorax:** urgent insertion of underwater pleural drain (see p. 119).

7. **Haemothorax:** insertion of underwater pleural drain, and blood transfusion. Penetrating injuries may continue to bleed after the insertion of a chest drain. Thoracotomy is then required.

Renal Injuries

History

These are manifest by *haematuria* and/or *renal pain, occurring after closed or open trauma to the loin which may on occasions have been quite trivial*.

Examination

1. Inspection of the **abdomen** and **loins** for the presence of *local bruising or swelling*.

2. Routine examination of the remainder of the **urogenital system**.

3. **Inspection and microscopic examination of the urine** and instructions that it should be saved for inspection each day.

Management

Bed rest—complete.

Sedation with opiates if necessary.

Urgent IVU—certainly within the first 12 hours. The purpose of this is not so much to determine the damage to the affected kidney, but to ensure that the other kidney is present and functioning in case an emergency operation should be necessary. If no function is seen on the IVU, an arteriogram or scan should be performed to ascertain that there is a blood supply to the kidney.

Operative intervention. In general, this is undertaken only if:

1. There is *persistent gross bleeding*.
2. There is *disruption of the kidney* with a perinephric collection of blood and urine presenting a swelling in the loin.

In these circumstances *renal arteriography* should be undertaken beforehand, to define the vascular injury and estimate whether repair, partial nephrectomy, or total nephrectomy will be necessary.

A further IVU is obtained before the patient attends the follow-up outpatient clinic.

Ruptured Urethra and Bladder

History

Both injuries are usually associated with fracture of the bony pelvis. Occasionally ruptured urethra may occur from blunt injury to the perineum, or bladder injury from a blow to the lower abdomen. If there is a fracture of all four pubic rami, a rupture of the membranous urethra should be strongly suspected.

Examination

Indices of suspicion are:

1. Inability to pass urine.
2. Blood from the urethra, or haematuria.

Management

In addition to the general management of what may be a severe injury, do *not* attempt to pass a catheter, but:

1. Undertake urethrography; if urethra is intact, then
2. Pass a soft catheter and perform *cystography*.
3. A partial urethral tear should be treated by temporary suprapubic urinary diversion.
4. A complete urethral rupture should be treated by suprapubic urinary diversion and the tear should be bridged by a urethral catheter. If possible the urethral ends should be approximated by drawing the prostate down onto the perineal diaphragm by sutures or traction.
5. A bladder tear should be repaired as soon as possible with adequate drainage of the suprapubic space.

Abdominal Injury

Both closed and penetrating abdominal injury are on the increase.

Closed injury

History. Try and find out exactly what happened. Sometimes this can be helpful in deciding how likely a closed injury is. Shoulder tip pain is often a pointer to rupture of spleen or liver.

Examination. Look for bruising, fractured lower ribs. Tenderness and guarding may be present but can be trivial; an unconscious patient may be unable to respond.

Special investigations. In instances of doubt, peritoneal lavage must be done. Under local anaesthesia a 1.5 cm incision is made just below the umbilicus and the peritoneum freed of surrounding fat. A dialysis catheter is then inserted by careful puncture into the peritoneal cavity and directed downwards. 0.5 litres of warm saline solution is run in and immediately drained out. Heavy blood staining, bile or gut content means laparotomy must be done. Light blood staining (less than 10 000 cells per ml) is compatible with retroperitoneal injury. Clear fluid almost certainly excludes serious intraperitoneal injury, but send it off for an amylase content. If operation is not immediately indicated, place the patient on hourly recordings of pulse and blood pressure.

Penetrating injury

Try and get a history of the weapon used—this will influence a decision about exploration or not: violent assault with a sharp kitchen knife and gunshot wounds are indication for exploration. The physical examination includes:

1. Signs of shock.
2. Evidence of intraperitoneal injury in the form of obvious venous ooze, bowel content or intraabdominal structures—bowel or omentum—visible in the wound.

In the absence of these cardinal signs there is often in stab wounds a policy of 'wait and see', but this does not apply to gunshot wounds.

Table 9

% body area burned	Age (yr.)							
	0-4	5-9	10-14	15-19	20-24	25-29	30-34	35-3⁹
93+	1	1	1	1	1	1	1	1
88-92	.9	.9	.9	.9	1	1	1	1
83-87	.9	.9	.9	.9	.9	.9	1	1
78-82	.8	.8	.8	.8	.9	.9	.9	.9
73-77	.7	.7	.8	.8	.8	.8	.9	.9
68-72	.6	.6	.7	.7	.7	.8	.8	.8
63-67	.5	.5	.6	.6	.6	.7	.7	.8
58-62	.4	.4	.4	.5	.5	.6	.6	.7
53-57	.3	.3	.3	.4	.4	.5	.5	.6
48-52	.2	.2	.3	.3	.3	.3	.4	.5
43-47	.2	.2	.2	.2	.2	.3	.3	.4
38-42	.1	.1	.1	.1	.2	.2	.2	.3
33-37	.1	.1	.1	.1	.1	.1	.2	.2
28-32	0	0	0	0	.1	.1	.1	.1
23-27	0	0	0	0	0	0	.1	.1
18-22	0	0	0	0	0	0	0	.1
13-17	0	0	0	0	0	0	0	0
8-12	0	0	0	0	0	0	0	0
3-7	0.	0	0	0	0	0	0	0
0-2	0	0	0	0	0	0	0	0

186

40-44	45-49	50-54	55-59	60-64	65-69	70-74	75-79	80+
1	1	1	1	1	1	1	1	1
1	1	1	1	1	1	1	1	1
1	1	1	1	1	1	1	1	1
1	1	1	1	1	1	1	1	1
.9	1	1	1	1	1	1	1	1
.9	.9	.9	1	1	1	1	1	1
.8	.9	.9	1	1	1	1	1	1
.7	.8	.9	.9	1	1	1	1	1
.7	.7	.8	.9	1	1	1	1	1
.6	.6	.7	.8	.9	1	1	1	1
.4	.5	.6	.7	.8	1	1	1	1
.3	.4	.5	.6	.8	.9	1	1	1
.3	.3	.4	.5	.7	.8	.9	1	1
.2	.2	.3	.4	.6	.7	.9	1	1
.1	.2	.2	.3	.4	.6	.7	.9	1
.1	.1	.1	.2	.3	.4	.6	.8	.9
0	.1	.1	.1	.2	.3	.5	.6	.7
0	0	.1	.1	.1	.2	.3	.5	.5
0	0	0	0	.1	.1	.2	.3	.4
0	0	0	0	0	.1	.1	.2	.2

If a decision is reached *not* to explore, repeated abdominal examination at hourly intervals and careful observation of pulse and blood pressure are essential. You should press for exploration if there are changes for the worse in either general or local signs.

Burns

There is an increasing tendency to refer burns to special units within your hospital, or at another hospital, where the accumulated experience of the staff can be used to handle the complicated problem of maintaining sterility and replacing damaged skin. Patients with extensive burns travel well in the early stages provided care is taken with fluid and electrolyte management. In the early phase it is important to do the following.

1. Make the distinction between a burn that is possibly survivable and one which is not. This is determined by combining age and extent of burn (disregarding the distinction between deep and superficial). The probability of death is shown in Table 9. It is clearly wrong to expend time and effort to prolong the agony of, say, a patient over 65–69 years with a burn of 68–72% of the body surface; however, every possible effort must be made for a 20–24 year old with the same area as he has at least a 30% chance of survival.

2. Burns over 15% in an adult and over 10% in children (i.e. less than 12 years of age) require intravenous therapy. Establish a line for the administration of fluids early, before hypovolaemia leads to vasoconstriction. Initial resuscitation is with Hartmann's solution and is guided by observation of *pulse*, *blood pressure*, *CVP*, and hourly *urine output*. The latter two are very useful when the arterial blood pressure may be difficult to take, and all patients burnt in excess of 25% should have a CVP line and urethral catheter inserted. The aim is to keep hourly urine output between 30 and 50 ml. In deep burns there is a risk of haemoglobin pigment released from haemolysed cells being swept to the kidney and producing tubular necrosis. Any patient who has a burn of greater than 30% full thickness, with darkening urine, or with progressive oliguria in spite of good circulation, should have 100 ml of 15% mannitol or 80 mg of frusemide administered to establish a diuresis.

3. Determine if there has been a respiratory burn by examining the throat of any patient who has been in a smoke-filled atmosphere

or has facial burns. Redness of the fauces indicates that over the ensuring 12–24 hours oedema of the larynx and bronchi may develop.

Local treatment

Partial thickness burns—treatment by: *exposure* in conditions of low humidity, bacterially-filtered, atmosphere; or by *closed dressings*, sulphamylon, or silver sulphadiazine.

Full thickness burns: (a) *very localised*—immediate excision and graft; (b) *more widespread*—treat as for partial thickness burn until about 10th day, when the whole extent of full thickness loss is evident: then split skin graft from patient. If donor skin is inadequate, cadaver allograft or porcine xenograft skin may be used as temporary cover.

Vascular Injuries

Laceration or transection of a major artery or vein, or traumatic occlusion of a major artery, both constitute clinical incidents in which time is of the essence. For details, see p. 134.

29. ORGAN TRANSPLANTATION
(See p. 11)

Not every hospital engages in organ (usually renal) allotransplantation, and nor is the general surgical house surgeon necessarily involved. On the other hand, renal autotransplantation is a technique that may be used in cases of renal artery stenosis, or when there has been loss of a substantial length of ureter from injury or other cause.

However, every hospital is a potential source of cadaveric donor kidneys and now other organs for allotransplantation. Potential donor patients are aged between 10 and 50 years, with apparently normal renal function, but with an inevitably lethal cerebral lesion. The latter may be caused by head injury, by spontaneous intracranial haemorrhage, as a result of cerebral anoxia from temporary cardiac arrest or as a result of a brain tumour. If such a patient should be on your service, contact the nearest Transplantation Unit after permission from your seniors. One preliminary requirement is that the patient cannot maintain spontaneous respiration and in the opinion of a senior staff member will never do so. The criteria for such 'brain death' vary from place to place, but should always be available in your hospital. It is usually at this time that permission of nearest relatives is secured for kidney donation, and in appropriate cases permission of the coroner. As a rule, a number of further investigations are made to determine the patient's suitability as a donor: tissue typing, blood urea concentration, and intravenous urogram. Special techniques are used to protect the organs against damage before the donor is declared dead, and during the 'warm ischaemia time' between when life support by respirator is withdrawn and the kidneys are removed and cooled. Each transplant unit has its own preferred regimen, but many use heparin and diuretics (frusemide or mannitol) prior to death. It is increasingly the practice to remove organs before respiratory support is withdrawn, so making 'warm ischaemia' time negligible.

30. 'MEDICAL' CONDITIONS

Because surgical patients are nowadays so often in the older age groups, many will be suffering from 'medical' conditions which may or may not bear on the diagnosis or on fitness for operation. As a general principle, if the condition directly impinges on the 'surgical' lesion or fitness for operation, it is fully investigated while the patient is in hospital, and a consultant opinion often obtained.

If on the other hand the 'medical' condition appears quite incidental, investigation is more limited, and most often it is sufficient to inform the patient's outside practitioner of the findings in the discharge letter, and leave it to his discretion to seek further advice or institute treatment.

It is important to appreciate that the amelioration of some 'medical' conditions may effect a profound reduction in operative risk.

It is also important to enquire into co-existent 'medical' conditions specifically from the point of view of drugs the patient is receiving or has received. Failure to be aware that certain drugs, e.g. steroids, have been taken is sometimes disastrous.

Any patient who has spent some time in hospital for medical or surgical investigation is likely to be unfit for a planned operation. If at all possible, such a patient should have a period of normal activity at home before non-urgent surgery is undertaken.

Diabetes Mellitus

1. If the patient is a known diabetic using insulin it is most important that before operation he be stabilised on *soluble* insulin.

2. If he is controlled by diet only, or by an oral hypoglycaemic agent, it *may* be necessary to use soluble insulin over the period of operation.

3. Diabetes is a very common disease and should always be thought of when the diagnosis is at all obscure, whatever the system apparently involved. Too often the diagnosis is missed because it has not been specifically sought: the reliability of the routine ward urine test is doubtful.

4. Serious illness, such as sepsis, and the use of high carbohydrate feeding regimens (p. 98) may give rise to problems of control. Two principles are used:

(a) sliding scale administration.

(b) continuous infusions.

5. Glucose may be measured either in the urine or in blood. Urine is less reliable and control of glucose aims to keep urinary glucose down to 'zero or trace' as measured by dipstick. A sliding scale is used for insulin administration viz:

0 – trace	0
¼ %	4 units
½ %	8 units
1%	12 units
2%	16 units

The insulin is administered subcutaneously and urine tested 6 hourly.

6. Glucose homeostasis is more easily achieved by measurement of blood glucose concentration. The Ames Dextrostix, when correctly used, will give a glucose concentration with an accuracy of +15% or 0.5 mmol/l when read on a Glucochek machine or an Ames

191

meter. These meters depend on the change in density of colour on the reagent pad of the Dextrostix after it has been in contact with blood for exactly 60 seconds. Blood glucose homeostasis in this situation is achieved using either continuous intravenous or subcutaneous *neutral* insulin delivered by a small-volume pump. The subcutaneous route is not suitable for a patient who is hypovolaemic as absorption may be irregular. The patient is started on 1 unit of insulin per hour and blood glucose concentration measured hourly, the rate of insulin infusion being adjusted to maintain the blood glucose concentration between 5–8 mmol/l. Two important points are:

(a) if the glucose concentration is falling, the insulin infusion should be turned down but not *off*, and

(b) the insulin requirements will rise if complications or surgery (e.g. sepsis) ensue.

These simple measures will deal with most situations. If there is diabetic ketoacidosis seek help unless you are very experienced.

Hypertension

1. Hypertension *per se* in the absence of cardiac failure gives rise to few difficulties during or after operation, provided any treatment which the patient normally receives is maintained.

2. It is most important that the anaesthetist is made fully aware in good time of any and all treatment for hypertension.

3. With modern drugs more problems arise from the withdrawal or modification of treatment than from continuing the normal regimen.

4. Nevertheless the patient on antihypertensive treatment is likely to have lost normal haemodynamic reflexes. Therefore, very accurate fluid balance to avoid depletion or overload is essential.

Adrenal Corticoids and ACTH
(See also p. 101)

These are used today in a wide variety of probable and improbable situations—to name but a few in the former group: rheumatoid arthritis, ulcerative colitis, 'collagen' disorders, anaemias, liver disease, asthma. Their significance with respect to surgery is:

1. They may *precipitate* a surgical situation or mask its onset, e.g. perforation or bleeding from a peptic ulcer.

2. Under conditions of stress such as *operation* the normal pituitary–adrenal response may be so suppressed that relative adrenal insufficiency exists with the production of dramatic *arterial hypotension*.

The tests for pituitary–adrenal suppression are at present too elaborate for routine use. Thus it is *vital* to any person receiving, or who has recently received (within the past year), these drugs that added systemic corticoids be given over the period of operation.

Anticoagulants

Many patients receive oral anticoagulant therapy, e.g. after cardiac valve replacement. This may become significant:

1. When bleeding occurs, such as into the urinary or gastrointestinal tract or into the tissues. Fresh frozen plasma and vitamin K 20 mg IM should be given. Intravenous vitamin K is no more effective, but may produce side-effects.

2. When a planned operation is to take place. A cardiologist should be consulted. Either the oral anticoagulant should be stopped at least five days before operation and a preoperative test should confirm a normal clotting mechanism, or it may be desirable to substitute heparin during the operative period.

3. When a surgical emergency requiring immediate operation arises. A difficult choice has to be made between reversing the oral anticoagulant with fresh frozen plasma and vitamin K with the potential danger of thrombosis or operating without such reversal which may in many instances prove to be quite safe.

The use of subcutaneous heparin for the prevention of thrombosis is now widespread. Its place is still not generally agreed. The surgeon should be informed whenever subcutaneous heparin has been given because many believe firmly that it contributes to postoperative oozing and even bleeding.

Jaundice

Drugs, too numerous to list, can produce cholestatic jaundice that may mimic extra-hepatic biliary obstruction. Postoperative jaundice may have a surgical or infective basis, and in minor degrees is a worrying associate of total parenteral nutrition, but may also occur from the use of halogenated hydrocarbon anaesthetic agents or at a later time from viral hepatitis. It nevertheless remains commoner for the physician to manage patients with extra-hepatic biliary tract obstruction medically, than it is for the surgeon to make the converse mistake.

Gout

This is a common condition. An acute attack is frequently precipitated by an operation and this may lead to the diagnosis being made for the first time.

The majority of patients with known gout will be on allopurinol and require no special treatment. Those not receiving allopurinol should be given this at a dose of 300 mg daily or a nonsteroidal anti-inflammatory drug (e.g. indomethacin 50–100 mg 6 hourly).

Chronic Respiratory Disease

This is common in those presenting for operation and most frequently is of the type broadly described as obstructive airways disease. Usually, much can be done to improve respiratory function especially before a planned operation. Patients with respiratory disease should usually be admitted several days earlier for elective surgery.

1. Stop the patient smoking if possible.
2. Choose the summer months for operation.
3. Reduce airways obstruction and sputum retention by an inhaled bronchodilator.
4. Encourage intensive physiotherapy in the form of breathing exercises, and sometimes postural drainage.
5. Consult with an experienced anaesthetist regarding the most appropriate anaesthetic—local, regional or general.

(See also p. 103).

Heart Disease

Myocardial infarction in the past, or chronic angina of effort do not necessarily render planned surgery dangerous. However, *recent* myocardial infarction adds greatly to the risks and no elective surgery should be done within three months and preferably not within six months of such an event. The risk is also high in patients with *unstable angina* and these should seldom if ever undergo elective surgery. Beware of patients who require surgery as a consequence of recent myocardial infarction (retention of urine from diuretics; peripheral arterial embolus; peripheral arterial or deep venous thrombosis).

The risk of other forms of heart disease is usually proportional to the degree of exercise intolerance. However, beware also uncontrolled dysrhythmia and the stenotic valvular lesion, especially when substantial blood loss may occur.

Any patient with bradycardia should be referred to a cardiologist for an opinion as to preoperative pacing.

31. INNER CITY PATIENTS

Those who work in inner city hospitals in the 1980's are likely to come across distinct groups of patients who will present with real or simulated surgical emergencies.

Munchausen Syndrome

This term, originally coined by Richard Asher, describes a patient whose history is so dramatic that it is either compelling, impossible or both (e.g. the original patient had had his many abdominal operations in a Japanese prisoner of war camp and his abdomen closed with string from Red Cross parcels), and whose signs are real but often out of tune with his/her demeanour. Though obviously not addicts, they frequently welcome opiates; are shifty about personal background; demanding of attention; and likely to take their own discharge. The houseman's job is to be aware of this problem and if a previous hospital admission is quoted to follow that up urgently (see p. 4). Their importance is that they must be distinguished from real *surgical* emergencies.

195

Opiate Addiction

The usual causes of surgical admission are:

1. Superficial or deep venous thrombosis, often with a septic element;
2. Subcutaneous sepsis.

Both require treatment on their merits. However, do not look for compliance or gratitude in these patients—they are interested in survival and where the next 'fix' is coming from. Referral to social workers and addiction centres is routine but rarely effective.

Rough Sleepers

All cities have a population of those who are 'of no fixed abode'. They get septic complications and hypothermia, both of which require treatment. They are usually keen to get out and back to their usual domicile.

32. FORENSIC PROBLEMS

House Surgeons rarely encounter situations with legal overtones which are so acute that they are unable to get advice from their seniors which should always be obtained. It is worth realising that a lack of expedition and of suspicion on the part of the House Surgeon may embarrass future legal manouevres to help the patient or to see that justice is done. House Surgeons must realise that in each situation the management of the patient must be placed before any broader societal considerations or responsibilities that may be thrust upon them by police or social workers who are interested in the case.

In all instances make written notes, preferably *pari passu* with the happening. Written notes may be augmented by good quality, well-lighted, black and white or colour photography. The names of witnesses should always be recorded in the patient's notes and any relevant timings should be recorded too.

Suspicious Circumstances

Road traffic accidents, in which either the driver or a pedestrian is injured may be associated with alcohol or drug abuse.

Child abuse is a not uncommon problem nowadays and unless the House Surgeon is on the ball, the abused child may be allowed home to be further damaged, perhaps fatally.

Cases of physical assault and of **alleged sexual interference** also come into Casualty Departments.

Road Traffic Accidents

At least 20 people are likely to die each day on the roads in the U.K. and many more will be injured. Many of the injured will be removed by ambulance and brought to hospital where the first opportunity for them to be examined by a doctor will occur. Most are 'real' road traffic accidents but occasionally a road traffic accident may be staged as a deliberate attempt to conceal an assault, a homicide or a suicide.

In Britain the putative driver involved in a road traffic accident is subject to the drink and driving provisions of the Road Traffic Act, 1972, and similar rules are in force elsewhere. The police may require the driver to have his blood alcohol estimated. Obtaining the specimens for this is a police matter. However, the House Surgeon must protect his patient's (and his own!) interests and should always try to obtain blood for alcohol estimation, particularly in an unconscious patient; a low blood alcohol may have a positive effect by protecting the patient from unwarranted prosecution. A blood alcohol level determined in an unconscious patient can only be used to assist in *medical management* unless the patient gives consent subsequently.

Any pedestrian injured or killed in a road traffic accident should also have his blood analysed for alcohol as a protection for the motorist.

Careful notes must be made of the time the casualty was brought to hospital and the time that the House Surgeon first saw and examined the patient. The state of the patient on arrival, whether conscious, unconscious, disorientated or rational, did they have any other injuries and careful details of measurements of all injuries should be made and written down. Photographs should be taken of injuries, insofar as it is possible, but in particular disfiguring facial injuries which are likely to be the subject of litigation at a later date should be photographed both before and after immediate surgical treatment.

197

Child Abuse

Child abuse may consist of physical injury when injury was inflicted or not knowingly prevented by a person having custody or care of the child. This includes cases where poisonous or noxious substances have been administered to a child and physical neglect when the child has been exposed to cold or starvation. Emotional or mental abuse is a further category and children so suffering may present as a 'failure to thrive'. It must be stressed that if one sibling in a house is suspected of suffering abuse, it is always advisable that the other children in the house should be examined.

The diagnosis is made by being suspicious and then carefully examining the child. Suspicions should always be aroused if injuries are incompatible with history or if the interval between the accident and reporting is prolonged. Good records must be kept of the time the child was examined, who brought the child to the doctor, what history was given by the parents and what history was given, if one was available, from the child. A full physical examination and urinalysis (especially for blood) must be made and photographs should be taken of any bruises. If the child is bruised and has injuries, X-rays of ribs, spine, limbs and head should always be taken to identify recent or old fractures which may indicate the time scale of the problem. It is useful to screen for clotting disorders.

If there is a reasonable doubt that the injuries are not purely accidental, the child should be admitted forthwith to the Paediatric Department. After this a senior colleague must be consulted, the Register/Index of Non-Accidental Injuries is interrogated and the Designated Nursing Staff/Social Worker informed. All Health Authorities in the United Kingdom have published policies for the management of non-accidental injuries to children whereby the police and the Social Services Department are involved and a case conference called. Usually by this stage the House Surgeon will have nothing further to do other than to report the findings that were apparent when the child was brought to hospital. Similar rules apply elsewhere.

Where other children are involved in the household, it may be necessary to make immediate arrangements for them to be examined and protected. In such cases it is best to have the child occupied and supervised by the nurses in hospital while you go elsewhere and alert your senior colleagues, the designated nursing staff and the Social

198

Services Department about the problem. The Social Services Department has the statutory obligation to place all the children in a protected environment.

Assault

Any medical practitioner may find himself called upon to examine a person who has sustained an injury of some nature and he may, at a later date, be required to report upon the injury and its possible sequelae either in criminal proceedings or in pursuit of a civil claim for compensation. The incidence of violence in the United Kingdom and elsewhere is increasing; cases of injury are now commonplace at football matches and similar sporting gatherings, including riots, and these cases may come under the management of a House Surgeon at any time.

Other injuries that are important include firearm injuries and stab wounds. The important role of the House Surgeon is in the correct recording of information, particularly when the patient first presents. Wounds are best divided into five categories: bruises, abrasions, lacerations, incisions and stab wounds, and each of these must be measured and described carefully. If possible the description should be aided by photographs. The colour of the bruises is important because this gives some indication of the time that they have been present. Scalds and burns are also wounds that may have been inflicted upon a person and careful details of their extent and their depth is vital. In the case of a minor, the written consent of a parent, guardian or close relation should be obtained before such a detailed examination is carried out. However, should such a person not be immediately available, the House Surgeon's responsibilities lie with the patient whom he must treat. The police are responsible for the collection of evidence and will ordinarily provide their own doctor who is specially trained in forensic medicine. The police may require the clothing for forensic examination because it may be important evidence. If it has to be removed in a hurry, the House Surgeon should ensure that it is taken off with as little damage as possible and that all stains, either wet or dry, and foreign substances such as mud, grass or dust that are on it are preserved. The clothing is put in a clean paper or plastic bag for scientific examination.

Physical examination of the assaulted person should include measurements of their height and weight which are of considerable practicality in assault between men in violent fighting. The following points should be sought and recorded:

1. The situation, number and type of wounds.
2. The size, shape, depth and direction of the wounds.
3. The condition at the edges, the ends and the base.
4. Any foreign bodies attached or embedded in the wounds.
5. Observations on haemorrhage, its source and volume.

In addition to these observations, routine observations of vital signs, particularly of the cardiovascular system, pulse, blood pressure, heart sounds, respiratory rate, and of the central nervous system, level of consciousness, etc., should be made.

It is worth recording these findings in great detail and making clear, simple diagrams and measurements of all wounds. Blood for alcohol levels or drugs should be obtained if there is any suggestion of alcohol or drug abuse. Photography is very valuable in cases of wounding; it is not simply to save making accurate notes but rather to amplify them and to provide refreshment to one's memory when evidence about the incident is required. Photographs have an evidential value of their own, provided safeguards are taken in their developing and printing. Many Casualty Departments nowadays have Polaroid cameras which will allow quick shots of the wounds to be taken. If the Casualty Department staff are doing this themselves they are well advised always to stick an adhesive metal tape with the name of the patient and the date on to the patient before the photograph is taken. In many cases of wounding, the police will wish to take their own photographs. This is not of direct concern to the House Surgeon, provided it does not in any way compromise the clinical care of the patient. However, the police must obtain the patient's consent before the collection of any photographs or blood samples etc.

Rape and Sexual Assault

It must be stressed that the victim of sexual assault is a patient first and foremost and must be treated as such.

If a female alleges a heterosexual assault it is best to assume at the beginning of the interview that rape has been committed. Females may present at hospital initially with minor stories of abdominal pain, trivial injuries or bruising and, after admission may allege that they have been the subject of a sexual assault. Ordinarily, such allegations should alert the nursing and medical staff who then report the matter to the police who will produce their own medical expert to examine the patient. In many cities there are also special centres for victims of rape or sexual assault. The House Surgeon may be caught out if he or she has already started to examine a patient who in the course of examination says that they have been the victim of a sexual assault. In these circumstances, the House Surgeon is best advised to desist from further examination and to take every possible step to ensure the patient's situation is not altered until a more adequate medical examination can be carried out by an expert. In particular, the nurses should not be allowed to wash or shower such a patient and all clothing from the patient should be carefully collected together and stored in brown paper or plastic bags.

Victims of sexual assault or patients who allege sexual assault deserve considerable sympathy and understanding from the medical and nursing staff. They may have already been subjected to a horrifying intrusion into their privacy and the further examinations that are necessary for the legal process are no less harassing. Useful help in this crisis can be obtained in the U.K. from voluntary Victims Support Schemes who can send a counsellor to the victim (National Association of Victims Support Schemes, London SW9—Tel. 01-737 2010).

Sexual assault may result in serious injury requiring urgent surgical intervention, for instance a vaginal rupture. In these circumstances it is useful for the operating team to be aware of the requirements of evidence for the courts. These should include pubic hair combings (all the pubic hair should be saved in a clean dry container if the patient is to be shaved prior to surgery), swabs from any bite marks, an introital swab, a perineal swab and a high vaginal swab (which should be obtained after insertion of a sterile unlubricated speculum BEFORE any internal examination). In cases where buggery is alleged, rectal swabs are indicated. Saliva for secretor status and blood for group, alcohol and drugs are additional investigations.

APPENDIX I

Enzyme nomenclature

(Based on the recommendation of the International Union of Biochemistry.)

Official Name (other names or abbreviations in brackets)	Abbreviation
Acid phosphatase	ACP
Alkaline phosphatase	ALP
Amylase (diastase)	AMS
Aspartate transaminase	AST (AAT, SGOT)
Cholinesterase	CHS
Creatine kinase	CK
Lactate dehydrogenase	LD (LDH)
Lipase	LPS
Pepsin	PPS
Trypsin	TPS

APPENDIX II

SI System

The SI (Système International) unit is being progressively introduced into medicine, but it will be a generation before the old units are phased out. We give below the basic SI units, some of the derived SI units and their proper abbreviations, and the standard symbols for multiples of SI units. We also give conversion factors for some of the SI units which WHO* has recently recommended be introduced into medical practice.

Basic SI units and abbreviations

Length	metre	m
Mass	kilogram	kg
Time	second	s
Electric current	ampere	A
Thermodynamic temperature	kelvin	K
Luminous intensity	candela	cd
Amount of substance	mole	mol

* 'The SI for the health professions' WHO, Geneva, 1977.

Some derived SI units, abbreviations and definitions

Energy	joule (J)	$kg\ m^2 s^{-2}$
Force	newton (N)	$kg\ m\ s^{-2} = J\ m^{-1}$
Power	watt (W)	$kg\ m^2 s^{-3} = J\ s^{-1}$
Pressure	pascal (Pa)	$kg\ m^{-1}\ s^{-2} = N\ m^{-2}$
Electric charge	coulomb (C)	$A\ s$
Electric potential difference	volt (V)	$kg\ m^2\ s^{-3}\ A^{-1}$ $= J\ A^{-1}\ s^{-1}$
Electric resistance	ohm (Ω)	$kg\ m^2\ s^{-3}\ A^{-2} = V\ A^{-1}$
Electric conductance	siemens (S)	$kg^{-1}\ m^{-2}\ s^3\ A^2 = \Omega^{-1}$
Electric capacitance	farad (F)	$A^2\ s^4\ kg^{-1}\ m^{-2}$ $= A\ s\ V^{-1}$
Frequency	hertz (Hz)	s^{-1}
Area	square metre	m^2
Volume	cubic metre	m^3
Velocity	metre per second	$m\ s^{-1}$
Molality	mole per kilogram	$mol\ kg^{-1}$
Concentration	mole per cubic decimetre	$mol\ dm^{-3}$

Prefixes for SI units

Fraction	Prefix	Symbol	Multiple	Prefix	Symbol
10^{-1}	deci	d	10	deca	da
10^{-2}	centi	c	10^2	hecto	h
10^{-3}	milli	m	10^3	kilo	k
10^{-6}	micro	μ	10^6	mega	M
10^{-9}	nano	n	10^9	giga	G
10^{-12}	pico	p	10^{12}	tera	T
10^{-15}	femto	f			
10^{-18}	atto	a			

Interconversions from selected 'old' units to SI units

'Old unit'	Multiplication factor, 'old' to 'new'	SI unit
Calorie (kcal)	4.18	Joule (J)
Pressure (mmHg)	0.133	kiloPascal (kPa)
(torr)	0.133	kiloPascal (kPa)
(cm H_2O)	0.098	kiloPascal (kPa)
Radiation (rad)	0.01	Gray (Gy)
(roentgen)	2.58×10^{-4}	Coulomb/kg (C/kg)

APPENDIX III

Laboratory Reference Ranges

In most instances the reference ranges given have been obtained from the Institute of Medical and Veterinary Science, South Australia. Where possible, the data conform with the SI system of units.

Haematology

Packed cell volume (PCV, haematocrit)	
—Male	42–52%
—Female	37–47%
Haemoglobin	
—Male	13.5–18.0 g/dl
—Female	11.5–16.5 g/dl
Erythrocytes	
—Male	$4.6–6.2 \times 10^6/\mu l$
—Female	$4.2–5.4 \times 10^6/\mu l$
Reticulocytes	0.1–4.0%
Mean corpuscular volume (MCV)	80–96 fl
Mean corpuscular haemoglobin (MCH)	27.0–31.0 pg

Mean corpuscular haemoglobin concentration (MCHC)	30.0–34.0%
Sedimentation rate (ESR)—Westergren	
—Male	< 5 mm/h
—Female	< 7 mm/h
Platelets	150–350 × 10^3/µl
Leucocytes	
—total	4.0–10.0 × 10^3/µl
—neutrophils	2.5–7.5 × 10^3/µl
—lymphocytes	1.5–3.5 × 10^3/µl
—monocytes	200–800 × 10^3/µl
—eosinophils	40–440 × 10^3/µl
—plasma cells	occasional
—blast cells	nil
—promyelocytes	nil
—myelocytes	nil
Bleeding time	0.18–0.36 ks
Clotting time	0.24–0.60 ks
Prothrombin time (one stage)	10–12 s
Prothrombin activity	70–100%
Activated partial thromboplastin time	30–40 s
Thromboplastin screening test (Hicks-Pitney)	8–10 s
Plasma fibrinogen	180–480 mg/dl
Euglobulin clot lysis time	7.2–18 ks
Serum fibrin degradation products (fibrin related antigen)	< 8 mg/l
Serum iron	
—Male	13–36 µmol/l
—Female	12–31 µmol/l
Serum folate	3–20 µg/l
Serum vitamin B12	150–740 pmol/l

Clinical Chemistry—Venous Plasma Concentrations

Sodium	137–146 mmol/l
Potassium	4.0–5.5 mmol/l
Calcium	2.1–2.6 mmol/l
Magnesium	0.7–0.9 mmol/l

Copper	11–22 μmol/l
Iron	12–32 μmol/l
Zinc	12–21 μmol/l
Chloride	97–108 mmol/l
Bicarbonate	22–31 mmol/l
Phosphate	0.8–1.5 mmol/l
Lactate	< 2 mmol/l
Pyruvate	< 0.1 mmol/l
Urea	3–8 mmol/l
Creatinine	50–130 μmol/l
Uric Acid	120–500 μmol/l
Glucose	3.3–5.5 mmol/l
Cholesterol	4–8 mmol/l
Triglyceride	< 1.8 mmol/l
Bilirubin	2–20 mmol/l
Protein	
total	64–83 g/l
—albumin	37–52 g/l
—alpha 1 globulin	2–4 g/l
—alpha 2 globulin	4–8 g/l
—beta globulin	6–11 g/l
—gamma globulin	6–16 g/l
—fibrinogen	1.8–4.8 g/l
Osmolality	285–295 mosmol/kg
Ammonia	< 50 μmol/l

Clinical Chemistry—Arterial Blood or Plasma

pH	7.38–7.42 pH units
Hydrogen ion activity (H^+)	38–42 nmol/l
Plasma bicarbonate	22–31 mmol/l
CO_2 tension (p_ACO_2)	35–45 mmHg
O_2 tension (p_AO_2)	75–100 mmHg

Clinical Chemistry—Plasma Clearance Values

| Bromsulphthalein retention | < 5% in 45 min |
| Creatinine clearance | 90–180 ml/min |

Clinical Chemistry—Serum Enzymes

Acid Phosphatase (ACP)	0–13 i.u./l
Tartrate labile fraction	0–5 i.u./l
Alkaline Phosphatase (ALP)	10–75 i.u./l
Amylase (AMS)	70–300 i.u./l
Aspartate Transaminase (AST)	10–40 i.u./l
Creatine kinase (CK)	< 46 i.u./l at 30°C
Lactate dehydrogenase (LD)	120–280 i.u./l
Pseudocholinesterase	3.3–9.4 i.u./l

Clinical Chemistry—24-hour Urine Excretion

Sodium	100–200 mmol
Potassium	25–100 mmol
Calcium (normal diet)	0.8–8.0 mmol
Chloride	100–200 mmol
Phosphate	13–55 mmol
Urea	36 mmol
Urobilinogen	< 70 μmol
MHMA (VMA)	< 30 μmol
Catecholamines	
—total	< 600 nmol
—noradrenaline	< 300 nmol
—adrenaline	< 300 nmol
5-HIAA	< mol
Hydroxyproline	305 μmol
Amylase	200–3000 i.u.

Clinical Chemistry—72-hour Faeces

Fat	< 18 g

APPENDIX IV

Table for Predicting Normal Total Body Water (TBW),
Extracellular Water (ECW), Total Body
(Exchangeable) Na^+ and K^+
(after Skrabal *et al.*, Brit. Med. J. **2**: 37, 1973)

W = weight of patient in kg
H = height of patient in cm
A = age of patient in years

Male

TBW (ml)	$= 300W + 200H - 110A - 11300$
ECW (ml)	$= 100W + 200H - 23700$
Na^+ (mmol)	$= 14.2W + 16.2H - 2.6A - 800$
K^+ (mmol)	$= 23.0W + 20.6H - 12.0A - 1570$

Female

TBW (ml)	$= 230W + 105H - 17350$
ECW (ml)	$= 136W + 76H - 6000$
Na^+ (mmol)	$= 17.9W + 5.2H + 470$
K^+ (mmol)	$= 15.3W + 3.9H - 12.6A + 1200$

INDEX

210

212

213

214